THE GOOD SLEEP GUIDE FOR KIDS

The essential guide to solving your child's sleep problems, from ages 3 to 10

SAMMY MARGO,
MSc MCSP HPC MMACP AACP

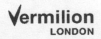

Vermilion
LONDON

1 3 5 7 9 10 8 6 4 2

Published in 2010 by Vermilion, an imprint of Ebury Publishing

Ebury Publishing is a Random House Group company

Copyright © Sammy Margo 2010

Sammy Margo has asserted her right to be identified as the author of this Work in accordance with the Copyright, Designs and Patents Act 1988.

The Random House Group Limited Reg. No. 954009

Addresses for companies within the Random House Group can be found at
www.rbooks.co.uk

A CIP catalogue record for this book
is available from the British Library

The Random House Group Limited supports The Forest Stewardship Council (FSC), the leading international forest certification organisation. All our titles that are printed on Greenpeace approved FSC certified paper carry the FSC logo. Our paper procurement policy can be found at
www.rbooks.co.uk/environment

Printed and bound in Great Britain by
CPI Mackays, Chatham, ME5 8TD

ISBN 9780091929695

Copies are available at special rates for bulk orders. Contact the sales development team on 020 7840 8487 for more information.

To buy books by your favourite authors and register for offers, visit www.rbooks.co.uk

This book is a work of non-fiction. The names of people in the case studies have been changed solely to protect the privacy of others.

Dedicated to my son, Daniel

Contents

Acknowledgements

I am extremely grateful to all the families who have shared their children with me. I have been privileged to have learned so much from their wisdom and understanding.

Thank you all for sharing.

Thanks to Gail Rebuck and Ed Victor, both of whom have made this book possible.

A huge thank you to Julia Kellaway for her insight, clarity, encouragement and fantastic editing. Thanks also to Naia Edwards for her cutting-edge research, and the rest of the team at Vermilion.

Thank you to The Chartered Society of Physiotherapy (CSP), which is working hard to 'improve the health of the nation'. I have been fortunate to work with a dedicated group of forward-thinking individuals. My special thanks to Prabh Salaman as well as Jennie Edmondson, Becky Darke, Becca Bryant and the rest of the team at the CSP. Thanks also to the CSP for supporting this book.

A great big thank you to all of my work colleagues who have let me get on with the book. Special thanks to Gayner, Tamasin, Karen, Steph, Naomi, Susie, Brad, Jade, Rhiann, Gemma, Julie and Vanessa. I would also like to thank Liz Mills and Susan Grossman for their professional guidance.

Thanks to my family, my special mum and dad who have always encouraged me to follow my dreams, my brother David and sisters Natalie and Caroline and their beautiful growing families who continue to give them all so much joy.

Thanks to my friends, especially those of you who are parents. I can't believe that we are talking about secondary schools for our kids and it feels like we just left school yesterday.

Finally a massive thank you to 'Efant' our special friend, to Isi for helping me through those long dark nights, and Daniel my son who is learning the 'art of sleep'.

Wishing you and your children 'sweet dreams'.

Introduction

'Good night, sleep tight' is what you say as you leave your child's bedroom, but how many of you know that it won't be long before your child gets out of bed or cries out, and how many of your children are actually getting a good night's sleep?

In fact, when was the last time you and your child had a really good night's sleep?

Difficulty with sleeping – whether it's getting to sleep, waking during the night or not sleeping for long enough – is one of the most common problems young children suffer from. If your child is having problems sleeping, the chances are that so are you. You may feel that you and your child will never get a decent rest again, but don't despair: with just a few simple changes your child's problems can be resolved. By following some of the practical advice in this book you can all enjoy a good night's sleep night after night.

Research shows that learning, performance at school, memory, mood, behaviour, social relationships, the risk of accidents and injuries, and weight all depend on a good night's sleep. Your child's sleep disturbance will also affect your health and well-being. So helping your child to sleep well not only benefits them but benefits the whole family.

Overall our children spend 40 per cent of their childhood asleep but, according to up to date research:

➤ 25 per cent of toddlers have problems settling down or waking up at night
➤ 14 per cent of children aged between 3 and 10 experience nightmares or night terrors
➤ 10 per cent of children sleepwalk
➤ 20 per cent of children have interrupted breathing problems in sleep such as sleep apnoea or snoring

We barely give it a moment's notice until our child can't sleep. Yet, based on the above statistics, a huge number of children are not getting enough sleep to feel properly rested and this is important when you understand the impact lack of sleep can have on a child.

As I explain later in this book, chronically sleep-deprived children often become chronically sleep-deprived adults. A few years ago I wrote *The Good Sleep Guide*, a practical no-nonsense handbook that tells you how to get a good night's sleep. In my work as a physiotherapist I see many people who suffer with sleep problems and I know the debilitating effects lack of sleep can cause. The sad thing is that many adults have been suffering from poor sleep since they were children. And yet I know that many sleep problems can be easily solved by following a few easy techniques – and this is true for children too. The earlier our children learn how to sleep well, the better it is for their health and their happiness. But, if we don't do anything about it, many children will grow into adults with insomnia or other chronic sleep problems, which will fundamentally affect their quality of life.

Over the last few decades, a great deal of research has been done into the causes and effects of sleeplessness on both adults and children and I have drawn from this research in this book.

But this is a practical guide too – much of the advice I give in this book for helping children to achieve better sleep is not theoretical but based on common sense, my experience as a physiotherapist and as a mother. Talking to clients about their children's sleep problems and discovering how and why children's sleep problems have changed over the years has helped too. It may sound obvious but one of the main reasons that children today are not getting the amount of sleep they need is because they are going to bed too late. The average child from the age of three and over goes to bed much later and gets less sleep than a child of even a generation ago. The reasons for this are various. With many of the preschool children I see, for example, both parents work and arrive home late. They keep their children up later so that they can spend some time with them before bedtime.

With older children, the reasons may be different. It has been estimated that, since the invention of the light bulb more than 100 years ago, people have lost over 500 hours of sleep a year. Today's primary schoolchildren not only have electric light in their bedrooms to keep them up after dark, but many also have televisions, computers, video games and mobile phones, which they play with long after they should have gone to sleep. Bedrooms used to be a place of calm and rest but have now turned into areas of high activity and places of play and stimuli. Many children now do not associate their bedrooms with places to wind down, relax and sleep.

Modern childhood is a very different world from the one we experienced ourselves. As parents (and I am the mother of a three-year-old boy) we all want the best for our children and this is no different from what our own parents wanted for us. What is different is the way we interpret what is best for our children. Whole industries are geared towards helping us make sure that children in the twenty-first century are not bored for a single minute during their waking hours and that they always have something to do. Activities are provided for our children at breakfast clubs before school starts and at after-school clubs at the end of the day. A great deal of emphasis is placed on helping our children become the brightest, the sportiest, the most musical or most beautiful, all of which involves our children being constantly entertained. Now many children don't know how to play by themselves and need to be permanently stimulated. This change from self-directed play is twinned with the fact that children today are leading increasingly sedentary lifestyles. If we cannot entertain our children ourselves – and many families with both parents working long hours cannot – then we allow our children to be entertained by the television or the computer or spending time on the mobile phone. With so many school playing fields being sold off, increasing health and safety issues at school limiting outdoor play, and parents less willing than their own parents were 20 years ago to allow their children to play outside for fear of 'stranger danger', the opportunities for physical activity are much fewer for a lot of young children today. The result is that our children are overstimulated, overworked and overcommitted at the same time as being underexercised, so it is hardly surprising that it takes our children time to wind down, switch off and finally go to sleep.

The reality is that in the fast-paced, multitasking, activity driven society we live in, we often find we don't have time to do things properly and we find short cuts. There's no time to cook properly, so we buy fast foods and ready-made meals that are quick, cheap and convenient but not healthy; there's no time to spend playing with our children and helping them unwind, and not enough time to give thought to our children's sleep patterns. We are not ensuring that our children get as much out of their sleeping hours as their waking hours or that they get the right amount of sleep. Yet making sure your child gets enough sleep is just as important to their health and well-being as paying attention to what they are doing during the day.

This book is not designed as a one-size-fits-all rulebook to sleep. Every child is different and every family works differently too so you will need to tailor the advice you find here to suit your child's and your own particular needs. But this book is designed to help you understand how much sleep your child needs to be healthy and provide practical information and suggestions for ways to achieve it. There are tips on every aspect of sleep from bedtime rituals and the bedroom environment to eating the right food before bedtime so I hope that before long you can wish your child 'Good night' as you turn out the light and know that they will get it.

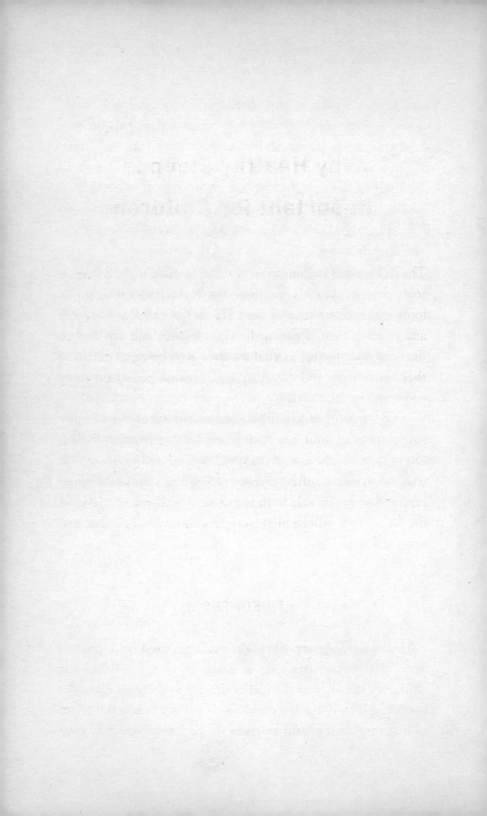

ONE

Why Healthy Sleep is Important for Children

The first step to helping your child get a good night's sleep is to understand why it's important. In this chapter I'm going to look at the different ways sleep affects our children's growth and development between the ages of three and ten and to discover that it's just as vital for their well-being as ensuring they eat healthy and satisfying foods, drink plenty of water and take regular exercise.

The benefits of a healthy night's sleep are obvious to any parent whose child has had a few late or broken nights. Depending on the age of the child, a tired child is slower to respond to things, often grumpy or liable to tears and temper tantrums, and less able to concentrate. A well-rested child, on the other hand, will be bright-eyed and bushy-tailed, alert and ready for action.

TIREDNESS

However old they are, all children will get tired from time to time, and this is perfectly normal. In fact, we want our children to be tired at the end of the day so that it is easier for them to get to sleep. If a child isn't tired when you put them to bed they won't want to go to sleep. Knowing when your child is tired and putting them to bed at the right time are key to helping your child achieve a healthy night's sleep. This isn't always easy. Some toddlers and young children will go to great lengths to be allowed to stay up and hide the fact that they're tired so they don't miss out on the action.

Sometimes children will show signs of being tired before their normal bedtime and you may think it is too early to put them to bed. It isn't. If you ignore the signs that your child is tired and keep them up, or if your child is not getting enough sleep, they are in danger of becoming overtired. Ironically, a child who is overtired is likely to become more active or hyperactive as time goes on, and to find going to sleep more difficult, even though they desperately need sleep. When children become overtired they may be too stimulated or wired to fall asleep.

Your Child's Sleepy Signs

A Tired Child

➤ Rubs their eyes or pulls their ears

➤ Yawns

➤ Becomes quieter

➤ Prefers slower activities, such as watching TV, to running around

➤ Sucks their thumb or finger or, if they use one, sucks a dummy

An Overtired Child

➤ Fusses, whines and becomes generally more irritable

➤ Is more prone than usual to tantrums and crying

➤ Is impatient

➤ Is clumsy

➤ Can become hyperactive

For your child to fall asleep quickly and easily at bedtime, and to enjoy a night of quality sleep, your child needs to be healthily tired at the end of the day but not overtired.

What makes a child tired, how much tiredness affects them and how much sleep they need varies for each individual, just as it does in adults. The reasons also vary according to the age of the child. Some of the most common causes of tiredness include: not enough sleep; lack of physical exercise; and lack of quality food.

NOT ENOUGH SLEEP

Preschool children aged three to five typically need between ten and twelve hours' sleep a day. Many children in this age group get tired during the day and need a nap to recharge their batteries. Watch out for signs that your child is tired. If your child has stopped having daytime naps, then make sure that they have quiet times during the day where they can rest and regain their energy.

The recommended amount of sleep for children aged between five and ten is about ten hours. It can be difficult to find out how much sleep your child is getting at this stage because they may lie awake for a long time after you've turned out the light. If you think your child is getting less than 10 hours' sleep at night, and is tired because they're not getting enough sleep, you need to find out why. Perhaps your child is being kept awake by his siblings? Does your child snore or have other breathing problems? These too could keep him awake.

Could your child be kept awake through anxiety? Talk to your child and encourage him to share his worries with you. It's important to choose the right time to talk to your child. Before bedtime may not be the best time to talk to him as it could remind him of his fear. Instead, find a quiet time during the day – perhaps on the way home from school – and try to get to the bottom of his anxieties then. Reassuring words from you will help to create the feeling of security he needs in order to get to sleep.

LACK OF PHYSICAL EXERCISE

Being physically active is an essential part of a healthy lifestyle and the tiredness that results from it contributes to promoting healthy sleep. Younger children tend to have bursts of energy in which they run around and are very active for a short time until they're exhausted. Having worn themselves out they stop for a while until their energy is restored and more activity follows. This pattern is repeated throughout the day until bedtime, when you hope that, tired out, they will fall asleep quickly.

For older children, physical exercise is just as important but unfortunately many children over the age of five are now getting less physical exercise than they should. According to research, only one in five parents know how much time children need to spend exercising a day. Ideally, children should be doing at least an hour of moderate physical exercise daily, which may be broken up into four fifteen-minute slots throughout the day. Parents should avoid their children 'binge exercising', where a surge of physical activity – such as an hour's gymnastics or swimming class – is followed by lots of sitting around. Young bodies aren't used to this kind of sudden change in activity and this can cause undue stresses and strains. The result is that about 25 per cent of my physiotherapy patients are children compared to only 1 per cent 20 years ago. Exercising little and often is the key to a healthier lifestyle and will better prepare kids for any classes they take, avoid potential injury, and help them achieve a healthy sleep every night.

LACK OF QUALITY FOOD

Being hungry and eating poor-quality food contributes to tiredness in children of all ages, but especially in preschool children who often become tired before meals as their blood sugar levels dip. Try giving healthy snacks such as a stick of cheese, or some fruit and vegetables between meals to keep their energy levels up and preparing home-cooked meals using fresh food. You can find out more about the effect of food on sleep in Chapter Ten. If you have problems getting your child to eat enough fruit and vegetables, you may want to consider giving them a course of vitamin supplements.

Children can also become tired and lethargic if they are not getting enough iron in their diet and they become anaemic. Iron, which builds the body's red blood cells, is fundamental to sleep and studies show that there is a strong link between iron deficiencies and sleep disturbances in childhood. Iron can be found in foods such as oily fish, eggs, green vegetables and iron-fortified cereals to name a few. Vitamin C helps the body to absorb iron so eating fruit rich in vitamin C, such as kiwi fruit and oranges, is a good idea too.

SLEEP AND YOUR CHILD'S HEALTH

Being normally tired is a necessary part of the sleep process. But tiredness that is caused by a persistent lack of sleep can have serious consequences for our children and result in their bodies not being able to develop normally. It is difficult to overestimate the effect that lack of sleep has on a child's temperament and physical development, and how it affects their sleeping patterns in later life; chronically sleep-deprived children become chronically sleep-deprived adults. This section explores the way in which sleep – or the lack of it – affects our children's health and development.

SLEEP AND YOUR CHILD'S IMMUNE SYSTEM

The health of both adults and children depends on the effectiveness of the immune system. The immune system is a network of cells, tissues and organs that is responsible for fighting off disease and protecting us from illness. So it's really important to make sure we keep our immune system as strong as possible. This is especially true for children whose immune system is developing and more vulnerable to infections.

Studies have shown that lack of sleep increases levels of a hormone called cortisol that weakens the body's immune system, making it less able to fight disease. Getting the right amount of sleep is one way to help strengthen the immune system to keep our children as physically healthy as possible and to give them the best chance of fighting off germs.

Tiredness is often a symptom of being ill. Young children catch coughs and colds frequently, especially once they start nursery or primary school and are in close contact with other children – and other children's germs! These infections can lay your child low for a couple of days and leave them feeling tired and lacking in energy. This tiredness usually passes quickly and disappears with the other symptoms of the illness. However, if your child feels persistently tired, or if being tired prevents your child from taking part in their ordinary activities, it is important to see your GP.

SLEEP AND YOUR CHILD'S GROWTH

If you have ever looked at your child in the morning and thought to yourself that they seem to have grown overnight, you are not imagining things. The human growth hormone (HGH), responsible for determining height and bone size during puberty, is secreted by the pituitary gland during sleep. The more sleep a child gets, the greater the production of this growth hormone and the greater the body's ability to develop to its full height. Although HGH is produced throughout our lives to regulate the body's metabolism, it reaches its highest levels during adolescence and is particularly important to the development of young bodies during that time. The right amount of quality sleep is vital for children to grow up big and strong.

Conversely, lack of sleep may stunt your child's growth. Researchers at the University of Philadelphia conducted a study in which they compared the sleep patterns in young children from New Zealand and India in 2008. The research revealed that the children from India received approximately two hours' less sleep every night than the children from New Zealand and that this had a harmful affect on their growth.

GROWTH SPURTS

The growth rate during a child's first year of life is astonishing – on average, babies grow 25 centimetres (10 inches) in length and triple their birthweight by their first birthday. After this time their growth rate slows down. Growth rates accelerate again at puberty; before that children may experience long periods of not growing at all, and then have a sudden growth spurt. During these periods, children often feel very tired and need to sleep more.

SLEEP AND YOUR CHILD'S WEIGHT

Obesity in children – where children weigh at least 20 per cent more than they should for their height – is a problem that is causing more and more concern, not only in the UK but in many parts of the world. Your GP can advise you as to what is a healthy weight for your child as you may find it difficult to tell whether your child has temporary 'puppy fat' or is genuinely overweight. Your GP will check height and weight charts (known as centile charts) when assessing your child to see if they are overweight for their age.

In England, it is estimated that between a quarter and a third of children are overweight and doctors and health officials are very seriously worried about the impact this 'fat epidemic' will have on the health service in years to come. An obese person is predicted to live nine years less than a person of average weight and there is a dreadful possibility that today's young children might be the first generation for many decades not to live as long as their parents.

But what has sleep got to do with this? Studies have been conducted all over the world to look at the correlation between sleep and weight and they have shown strikingly similar results. In Japan, Canada and Australia studies on the sleep patterns of young children all showed that kids typically aged five and six who got less than eight hours' sleep had a 300 per cent higher rate of obesity than kids who slept a full ten hours. Studies by sleep scientists in the US found the same thing: children who sleep less are fatter than children who sleep more. In the UK, too, researchers at the University of Bristol found that, of the thousand people they studied, those individuals who spent less than eight hours sleeping had a greater likelihood of being heavier.

These studies are quite surprising. The natural thing to assume would be that the more hours a person is awake and being active, the more likely he is to be losing weight. But this is not the case. Why?

A number of experiments have revealed that sleep loss causes hormonal changes that increase the appetite. The hormone ghrelin, which signals hunger, is increased if you don't get enough sleep while at the same time the hormone that suppresses appetite, leptin, decreases. Furthermore, the stress hormone, cortisol, is increased with sleep loss; cortisol stimulates your body to make fat.

In the studies that were carried out, it was seen that not only did people who were sleep-deprived eat more as a result of their increased ghrelin levels, but they tended to eat more sweet and starchy foods, two food groups that convert easily into fat. On top of that, the production of HGH (human growth hormone), which is needed to help break down fat, is inhibited when the body lacks sleep and cannot function as well.

Dr Shahrad Taheri, whose work in the University of Bristol was responsible for a lot of these findings, found evidence that children as young as two years old may be in danger of becoming obese if they lose a lot of sleep.

Apart from these hormone shifts that occur with sleep deprivation, which increases the likelihood of your child gaining weight, logic also suggests that:

➤ the more hours your child is awake, the more time they have to fill with eating food
➤ the less sleep your child gets, the more tired they become and less inclined to take healthy exercise

➤ the more tired your child is, the more likely they are to crave comfort food

Obviously you should not expect your child to lose weight simply by sleeping. Providing your child with a sensible diet and making sure they get enough exercise are the two most important things you can do to ensure your child maintains a healthy weight. However, getting enough sleep certainly plays an important part in preventing too much weight gain.

SLEEP AND YOUR CHILD'S MOOD

The importance of making sure your child gets enough good sleep is not only to help maintain their physical health but their mental health too. Lots of parents will have experienced a child who becomes moody, irritable, grumpy and negative after a couple of late bedtimes or early mornings. It is still unclear why a lack of sleep causes irritability – although one theory is that it may have something to do with the body's production of cortisol (the stress hormone), which is increased with sleep loss. Whatever the reason, your child's usual good temper can easily be restored, provided they resume a normal healthy sleep routine.

More seriously, however, is if your child is persistently suffering from lack of sleep, as this may be an early sign of depression or other emotional disorder. Clinical depression, as distinct from the odd day of feeling blue, is known to affect about 2.5 per cent of children in the US and 2 per cent of children under 12 in the UK – rising to 5 per cent of teenagers. In 2008 research was carried out on 122 children aged between 7 and 11 who suffered from depression. Eighty-two per cent of these children said that they had problems sleeping.

These problems included difficulty with getting to sleep and worrying about not being able to sleep, shorter sleep times and waking during sleep.

Research is ongoing into whether lack of sleep can actually cause depression and mental illness in children and adults. Certainly there are those who believe that it can. Whatever the results of this research, it does seem clear that sleeping well contributes to a healthy mind as well as a healthy body.

SLEEP AND YOUR CHILD'S PERFORMANCE AT SCHOOL

Inadequate sleep can have a negative effect on how well your child does at school, both in the classroom and in the playground because it affects their cognitive abilities, such as memory and attention span, as well as their temperament.

Memory

A good night's sleep helps to improve the memory. Research has shown that even a short nap can help improve IQ levels. For some time scientists have known that the popular advice to 'sleep on it' in order to solve a problem did have some truth to it, but did not know exactly why it worked.

New research, however, using functional magnetic resonance imaging, which shows the parts of the brain that are active while someone is being tested, gives us a much better understanding of how sleep loss impairs a child's brain. The scans show that while you are asleep the brain becomes active at storing new memories and consolidating new information, particularly of things you have just been taught how to do. As well as that, the scans also show that after a period of sleep the part of the brain that controls speed and accuracy is more active, resulting in newly learned skills being performed more easily and automatically. Clearly then, children need more sleep than adults as they develop new skills and learn new things every day. While a child is asleep, all the information they have learned during the day is consolidated and shifted to a more efficient storage region in the brain.

Tests on the memory and attention of school-aged children have shown that those who get even one less hour of sleep than their peers perform less well. This is especially true when our children are at a stage in their lives where they are having to absorb a lot of new information, for example when they are starting school, learning to read for the first time and learning to write. During these times of intensive learning it is really important they get sufficient sleep. Well-rested children have an astonishing, sponge-like capacity for gaining and retaining new knowledge; the more a child learns during the day, the more they need to sleep at night, and the more they will learn during the next day. If your child is not getting enough sleep, then they will find it harder to remember how to perform new tasks.

Attention Deficit Hyperactivity Disorder (ADHD)

ADHD refers to a range of problem behaviours associated with poor attention span, including impulsiveness, inattentiveness and hyperactivity. About 3 per cent of school-age children in the UK, mostly boys, have been diagnosed with it and the effects of it usually prevent that child (and often the ones around him) from learning well and mixing in with other people. These behavioural problems are remarkably similar to the problems experienced by children who suffer from lack of sleep, and for this reason – and for the reason that these days we seem to be more keen to label children – many children are misdiagnosed with ADHD when in fact they are sleep-deprived.

Scientific studies have confirmed the link between sleep and behavioural problems. One study found that up to half the children tested with ADHD suffered from sleep complaints compared to just 7 per cent of other children. In another study, researchers at the University of Helsinki and the National Institute of Health and Welfare in Finland tested how long 280 7- and 8-year-old children slept and then compared the results to a series of tests designed to diagnose ADHD. They found that the children who got an average of less than eight hours' sleep a night had a higher chance of showing symptoms of ADHD. The findings from their study show that maintaining adequate sleep schedules for children is a key factor in preventing behavioural symptoms. They suggest, too, that part of the solution for dealing with behavioural problems may just be as simple as sorting out a child's sleep habits.

SLEEP AND YOUR CHILD'S RISK OF INJURY

Is your child accident prone? Is he always bumping into things or falling over and hurting himself? If so, one possibility is that he might not be getting enough sleep. Studies have been carried out in different countries including China, Italy and England that indicate that children under the age of 14 who do not get the recommended amount of sleep are more likely to be injured than children who sleep well. Although the amount of sleep a child needs varies a little according to age and for each individual, the Sleep Council in Britain recommends that toddlers sleep for around 12 hours a day and primary school children between 5 and 11 should normally have from 10 to 11½ hours sleep a night. The increased risk of injury for a child who isn't getting enough sleep is alarming – they are twice as likely to be hurt than children who are well rested, and in some surveys the findings are even greater: a survey in Italy showed that children who slept less than 10 hours a day had an 86 per cent increase in injury risk, particularly if they were boys.

TIME TO PUT SLEEP FIRST

If asked to write a list of the most essential things to provide for a child I suspect most people would put: healthy diet, warm and clean clothes, a roof over their heads, good exercise and education, but I wonder how many would include ensuring the child had enough good quality sleep? Sleep often comes low down the list of priorities, despite the fact that lack of sleep has such a big impact on a child both at school and at home. Children need a good night's sleep to perform properly academically, to feel better about life generally, to stay fit mentally and physically. So it's about time that we made sure that helping our children sleep healthily is a high priority on our list.

TWO

Understanding Sleep

For many years it was believed that nothing very much happened when we were asleep and that it was just a time when our bodies shut down for a few hours. We now know that our brains are actually very active during sleep. We also understand more about how sleep works, our body's need for sleep and the cycles of sleep in adults and children. This knowledge can help us to understand when and why our children wake during the night and to solve the sleep problem. It can also help us to work out what we can do to make sure our children get the right amount of sleep so that they can make the most of every day.

THE NIGHTLY SLEEP CYCLE

When our children go to sleep at night, they don't just fall instantly into a deep sleep and then wake up again ten hours later. What in fact happens during the course of the night – for both adults and children – is that we cycle back and forth into different levels or stages of light and deep sleep, and dream sleep. The sleep cycle in a full-term newborn baby is about an hour long, but this increases to 90–110 minutes by the time a baby reaches 3 months and stays like this for the rest of our lives. Every time your child comes out of one sleep cycle and before they enter another, a degree of awakening occurs. This means that about five times a night your child, although not properly awake, is in a very light sleep and vulnerable to waking up. But, while waking up in the night is natural, it is also natural for your child to go back to sleep without needing help from you.

Our sleep cycles are divided into two types of sleep: Non-REM sleep, which is divided into four stages (see below) and REM Sleep (Rapid Eye Movement sleep), when we do most of our dreaming. Different things happen to our bodies during each sleep stage, all of which are important.

In Non-REM sleep the blood supply to the body's muscles is increased, tissue growth and repair occur and important hormones are released for growth and development.

In REM sleep the brain becomes very active, with blood flow nearly doubling and the body increasing its manufacture of certain nerve proteins, the building blocks of the brain.

Learning to understand these sleep cycles can help your child to get better sleep. When your child is in a light sleep, it's particularly important to keep things quiet so as not to disturb them. When they are in a deep sleep they are harder to wake up, so this may be a good time if you need to get something from your child's room, as they will hardly be aware of what's happening and will go back to sleep easily.

NON-REM SLEEP

Stage 1

Once your child has settled down it should take them no more than 10–15 minutes to get off to sleep. For the first five to ten minutes after your child goes to sleep, they are in a very light or drowsy state of sleep. This is the time when you may well have to keep the noise down. The muscle activity slows down, though it is common to have hypnagogic startles, muscle contractions and twitches which immediately precede a sudden sensation of falling (this is common in adults too). If you were to observe your child at this stage you would see the eyes moving slowly under the eyelids but, although they are asleep, they can be easily woken up by any sudden noises in the house or other change in the environment, such as a light being switched on. Children who fight sleep may enter this first stage and then pull themselves back to being fully awake at the last minute just before they enter into stage 2 sleep.

Stage 2: Light Sleep

During this stage your child's body temperature decreases, the heart rate slows down and the eye movements stop. At the same time the brain waves become slower, with occasional bursts of rapid waves called sleep spindles. In light sleep your child is not woken up quite so easily, so you can carry on business nearly as normal although they are still not heavily asleep. This stage lasts about twenty minutes in adults and children over the age of three.

Stages 3 and 4: Deep Sleep

It can be very difficult to wake a child up during stages 3 and 4, which together are called deep sleep. During these stages of sleep, you can carry on as usual with minimal concern for waking your child but if your child is woken up then they are likely to take a few minutes to adjust to being awake and will feel groggy and disorientated. Make sure you give your child some time to come round.

While your child is in deep sleep there is no eye movement or muscle activity and blood flow decreases to the brain, going instead to muscles in other parts of the body and restoring physical energy. It is during this period that our immune functions increase and growth hormones are released, so it's very important for your child's physical development. It is also the time that children are most likely to experience bed-wetting, night terrors or sleepwalking (see Chapter Four for more on these conditions).

REM SLEEP: DREAM SLEEP

After being asleep for about 70–90 minutes your child will enter into the first REM (or Rapid Eye Movement) sleep, so called because, if you were to look at your child asleep, now you would see their eyes dart around under their eyelids. And if you were to listen to your child during this stage you would hear that their breathing was quick and shallow. The heart rate and blood pressure also increases and the limb muscles become paralysed.

REM sleep is sometimes referred to as dream sleep as this is when most of our dreams occur, although dreams can take place in other stages of sleep. Nightmares also happen while your child is in REM sleep. It is during this stage that the brain is actively working at processing emotions, relieving stress and consolidating memories of the day. It is also thought to be vital to learning, stimulating the brain regions used in learning and developing new skills. Because young children have so much new information to take in each day and to remember, this stage of sleep is particularly important for them. This is why toddlers and young children have considerably more dream sleep than adults. Toddlers spend approximately 50 per cent of their sleep in REM sleep – even unborn babies from six months' gestation have a period of REM sleep. By the age of three this drops to 33 per cent and by the ages of 10–14 children get the same amount of REM sleep as adults, which is about 25 per cent of their sleep.

The first sleep cycles each night contain comparatively short REM periods and long periods of deep sleep. As we go through the night, the period of active REM sleep becomes longer while the amount of time we spend in deep sleep becomes shorter. This explains why many children will sleep for quite a long period without waking up in the first half of the night but then have periods of frequent waking in the second half of the night. If your child is not sleeping for long enough, it means they are missing out on REM sleep, which is, as we've seen, so important for learning and developing new skills. A child that is woken up too early may also be mentally less sharp as a result of losing some of the mentally restorative REM sleep.

CIRCADIAN RHYTHMS

How do our bodies know when it is time to sleep? The answer is that, like all living creatures, we have cycles of daily activity called circadian rhythms (circadian is Latin for 'around a day').

These rhythms are controlled by our internal or biological clock that gives us cues for when the day begins and when it ends, making us feel awake and alert during the day and sleepy at bedtime. This clock actually runs on a 25-hour cycle but it resets itself each day based on exposure to light and dark, our mealtimes and our sleep times, which is why having a good bedtime ritual and a quiet dark place to sleep is so important. Lack of routines and haphazard nap or bedtimes can easily upset our body clocks.

The circadian cycle is controlled by a region of the brain known as the hypothalamus, which is the main area for establishing sleep patterns. When it receives signals about light and dark from the retina of the eye it transmits this to the pineal gland that is responsible for the production of the sleep hormone called melatonin. When it's light, melatonin production decreases so we wake up. Conversely, when it's dark melatonin production increases so the body begins to prepare for sleep. Interestingly, research has shown that prenatal exposure to high levels of cortisol (stress hormone) may affect the development of the area of the brain that deals with sleep patterns.

Our circadian rhythms only start developing at about six weeks old – until that time newborn babies often have night/day confusion, sleeping equally during the day and night. Gradually, after about six weeks, babies start to have a sense of night and day and, by three months, a baby should be sleeping more during the night than the day. Daytime sleep gradually decreases over the first three years of a child's life and most children by the age of four are no longer having a daytime nap.

HOW MUCH SLEEP DOES MY CHILD NEED?

The amount of sleep your child needs depends both on the age of your child and on the individual child itself. Not all children in a certain age group need to have exactly the same amount of sleep. For example, some children at the age of three, like my son, may need to sleep for a whole twelve hours to feel alert the next day, while other three-year-olds may only need ten hours to feel the same benefits.

Signs that your child is getting enough sleep:	Signs that your child is not getting enough sleep:
➤ happy during the day	➤ difficult to wake up in the morning
➤ physically active throughout the day	➤ falls asleep during the day
➤ seems alert and responsive all day	➤ has erratic behaviour during the day

SLEEP GUIDELINES

While it's true that each child is unique and has their own particular requirements, it is helpful to have a guideline for how much sleep a child needs. Most kids' sleep requirements do fall within a predictable range of hours based on their age. If your child is not regularly getting something near the amount of hours mentioned below, then they may be getting chronically overtired and sleep deprived, but don't worry, there are some easy ways to ensure your child gets enough sleep.

Age of child	Hours of sleep recommended	

3–5	10–12	• Average sleep needed is 10–12 hours per night, and it should take your child about 20 minutes to go to sleep. However, all children are different and some take longer to fall asleep. This is fine, as long as they're not distressed. (See page 39)
		• What time they go to sleep doesn't seem to matter as long as they consistently get 10–12 hours' sleep
		• Decide what works best for your family:
		  O Parents arrive home later in the evening? You may prefer to spend time with your children before they go to sleep so put them to bed later
		  O Early risers? Put your children to bed early
		• No matter what schedule you choose, remember is it vital that the bedtimes are consistent and that your child goes to bed at roughly the same time every night

5–9	10	• From this age onwards the amount of time your child needs to sleep decreases to about 10 hours a night • Your child will now be starting school, and will need to be up at a certain time in the morning to start getting ready

Age of child	Hours of sleep recommended	
5–9	10	• Factor the new bedtime into your and your child's lifestyle before they start school – you may need gradually to adjust the time your child goes to bed over the course of a few nights if your child's new bedtime will be significantly different
9–11	9½–10	• The pre-adolescent child usually needs about 9½–10 hours' sleep • This is actual sleep time! Not from the time you turn off the light • Your child should take about 20 minutes to get to sleep • Try to minimise distractions in the room so that televisions, computers and mobile phones are either switched off at bedtime or removed from your child's room entirely

It can be particularly difficult to make sure that your school-child gets enough sleep. While you are trying to make sure your child goes to bed early enough to feel rested in the morning and able to get the most out of school, suddenly there are so many other demands on your child's time. There's often homework for children to do as well as after-school clubs, sports and activities. Friends are asked over to play and to stay for tea and increasingly TV, computers, the Internet, video games and other media become more interesting to your child and claim more of their time. All of these things – especially watching TV just before bedtime – can make it difficult for your child to want to go to bed or to be able to get to sleep once they are under the covers. Nightmares and other disruptions to sleep are common, as well as feeling anxious about sleep and not getting enough sleep every night.

WHAT HAPPENS WHEN MY CHILD DOESN'T SLEEP?

As discussed above, many children do not get the amount of sleep they need, especially once they have started school and there are so many other more interesting and fun things to do than sleep! But sleep, as we know, is essential for the development of our children's minds and bodies in so many ways. While the odd night of broken sleep is not going to be of any serious consequence, persistent lack of sleep or poor sleep can lead to mood swings, behavioural problems such as hyperactivity, lack of concentration and poor memory, all of which affects children's learning ability at school.

Recent studies have suggested that while we are asleep is an important time for replenishing energy stores that have been used up during the day and which are needed for our cells to function. The less sleep your child has, the less time they have for building up their energy supplies, and also they have less time for the production of hormones, such as the growth hormone that is released while your child is asleep and is important not just for growth but also for processes like muscle repair.

Common Symptoms of Sleepless Nights are:

➤ difficulty getting up in the morning
➤ feeling sleepy throughout the day
➤ inability to concentrate
➤ constantly seeking stimulation and attention
➤ irritable, cranky
➤ slower to perform ordinary tasks
➤ more likely to bump into things and be accident-prone
➤ body takes longer to heal after injury
➤ exaggerated emotions
➤ dark circles under the eyes
➤ yawning
➤ less able to fight off illnesses owing to a weakened immune system
➤ lacking in energy

Not all of these symptoms may be present in your child. For example, according to the National Sleep Foundation in America, not every child who is not getting enough sleep will appear to be tired. Sometimes lack of sleep can make children hyperactive, causing them to be impulsive and inattentive. The suggestion is that children who don't get enough sleep need to create a stimulating environment to keep themselves awake, so that they can learn.

HOW LACK OF SLEEP AFFECTS YOUR CHILD'S SLEEP

Sleep begets sleep. The strange thing is that often the less children sleep and the more overtired they become, the harder it is for them to get to sleep – and when they do get to sleep they often don't sleep well. These children wake up frequently and suffer from other sleep problems such as nightmares, sleepwalking and night terrors. Having had a bad night's sleep causes both the child concerned and the rest of the family to feel irritable and stressed and therefore less likely to go easily to sleep the next night, making the vicious circle of sleeplessness difficult to break.

Children, of course, don't complain about being sleep-deprived – they don't know that's what they are. They're not old enough to understand that even getting one hour's sleep less a night than they should can have a tremendous negative impact on their health and well-being. It is up to the parents to make sure that their children are getting the right amount of sleep to meet their needs and, if not, to work out why not. In the next chapter, we will look at reasons why your child may not be getting the amount of sleep they need and whether your child has a sleep problem, and help you to find out whether you need to be doing more to help your child get a good night's sleep.

THREE

Why is My Child Not Getting a Good Night's Sleep?

The chances are that you are reading this book because you are worried that your child is not getting a good night's sleep. If so, you are not alone. Sleep deprivation is a very common problem in children, with an estimated 65 per cent at one time or another not getting the amount of sleep they need; teachers report that 10 per cent of schoolchildren fall asleep during class. So how do you know if your child is getting a good night's sleep or if they are deprived? Perhaps you think to yourself that it's normal that your child wakes up very early or doesn't go to sleep until late at night. Perhaps if you are tired and not getting enough sleep you think this is just an inevitable part of parenthood? Knowing whether your child is getting enough sleep can be difficult because, as I said in the last chapter, every child is different and their sleep needs are different. And it can be difficult to know whether your child is sleeping enough. The time that you put your child to bed is not necessarily the time that he goes to sleep.

IS MY CHILD SLEEP-DEPRIVED?

The first step to finding out whether your child is sleep-deprived is to look at the guide to the average amounts of sleep a child needs on pages 22–3 to find out how much sleep your child should be getting. Then, to help you find out further whether your child is getting enough healthy sleep, take a look at the quiz below:

Quiz

➤ Do you have to wake your child almost every morning?

➤ Does your child sleep in at weekends?

➤ Does your child get cranky, irritable, aggressive or very emotional during the day?

➤ Does your child have trouble concentrating during the day?

➤ Does your child fall asleep in the car often?

➤ Is your child hyperactive at a time when you would expect them to be tired?

➤ Does your child often nod off while watching TV?

➤ Does your child fall asleep at other times during the day?

➤ Does your child suck their thumb, finger or dummy at times other than bedtime?

➤ Does your child get irritable, bad-tempered or defiant towards the end of the day?

➤ Does your child wake frequently at night?

➤ On some nights, does your child fall asleep much earlier than their usual bedtime?

➤ Does your child take longer than 20 minutes to fall asleep?

If you answered yes to more than two of these questions, then your child is probably not getting enough healthy sleep at night and is sleep deprived. In other words, if your child can go to bed and fall asleep easily, wake up easily and not be tired during the day, then they're probably getting enough sleep. If your child finds it difficult to get to sleep and this is causing daytime problems, such as falling asleep during the day or not being able to concentrate properly, then they are sleep-deprived.

KEEP A SLEEP DIARY

If you are not sure about the answer to any of the questions in the quiz above, you may find it helpful to keep a sleep diary. This is a diary in which you note down information about how and when your child falls asleep over a particular amount of time, up to a week. Looking at this information will help you discover more about your child's sleep patterns and see whether there is a problem, and if there is, what it's likely to relate to.

On the next page is a form that you can photocopy to keep as a record of your child's sleep.

Sleep Diary

Date: _____

Total hours slept: _____

Times and lengths of naps: _____

Food. What did they eat? _____

    When did they eat? _____

Exercise. What did they do? _____

    When did they exercise? _____

What did they do before bed? _____

_____

What time did they go to bed in the evening? _____

    When did they settle? _____

Issues in settling: _____

    What did you do? _____

    How did it work? _____

Times and lengths of waking at nights: _____

    What did you do? _____

    How did it work? _____

Any other observations? _____

_____

_____

Next day. How is your child:

    Physically? _____

    Mentally? _____

    Emotionally? _____

Notes: _____

_____

_____

WHY IS MY CHILD SLEEP-DEPRIVED?

There are various reasons why your child may not be getting enough sleep but it is clear to me that one of the main reasons why sleep-deprivation in children is such a modern epidemic is the highly pressured, competitive society our children are now brought up in. Children and young people are often overstimulated, overscheduled, overworked and over-committed; therefore it is hardly surprising that they should become overtired. Additionally, children's bedrooms have become a place where mobile phones, TVs and video consoles are a common feature. This means that, instead of children going to their room to sleep, they spend their time watching TV, playing video games, texting their friends or surfing the Internet. Studies have shown that children with a TV in their room are likely to spend an additional five and a half hours watching it, time when they could – and should – have been asleep. In addition, if the computer or TV is in your child's bedroom, it's very difficult for you to monitor what they watch or have access to.

Chloe was given a mobile phone for her eighth birthday, after which time she seemed to spend far more time than usual in her bedroom. Her parents couldn't figure out why she was so exhausted until they received the first unexpectedly high phone bill, which showed that Chloe was on the phone until 2 a.m. and sometimes until 4 a.m. She had actually fallen asleep while on the phone to her friend then woken up in the night and turned it off. Her parents soon put a stop to her having a mobile phone in the bedroom!

SLEEP DEBT

If your child is not getting enough sleep, they will be accumulating what is called a sleep debt. A sleep debt can range from one night's very poor sleep to many days of not enough sleep and it needs to be paid off. So, if your child normally sleeps for 10 hours a night but only gets 8 hours, they should sleep for 12 hours the following day. However, if your child is regularly missing two hours' sleep a night, their sleep debt will become chronic and this can lead to poor mental and physical health. Research shows that many adolescents are racking up a two-hour deficit every weeknight – that means 10 extra hours of sleep are needed by each weekend, which leaves very little time for anything else. Even if your child can catch up by sleeping in, it's not a good idea. If they have a long lie-in on Saturday and Sunday, that means they probably won't be tired on Sunday evening, so they'll start the week off on the wrong foot. Instead, you should make sure your child goes to bed earlier and wakes up at the same time every day, including weekends and days off. Your child may complain that their bedtime is earlier than their friends' bedtimes and it's unfair that everyone else gets to stay up later. You will have to reassure your child that every child is different but that their bedtime is the right time for them because it keeps them healthy.

HOW DO YOU MAKE SURE YOUR CHILD GETS ENOUGH SLEEP?

The answer to this depends on the reasons behind your child's sleep-deprivation. The following quiz will help you assess what may be stopping your child from getting the healthy sleep they need and whether or not they have a sleep disorder.

Quiz: Do you have a healthy sleep strategy in place?

➤ Does your child go to bed at a different time each night depending on their daytime activities?

➤ Do you wait for your child to fall asleep before putting them to bed?

➤ Does your child go to bed later at weekends and have long lie-ins?

➤ Does your child watch TV or play video games or use the computer before going to bed, or fall asleep in front of the TV?

➤ Does your child take a mobile phone to bed with them?

➤ Does your child do less than an hour of exercise every day?

➤ Does your child exercise near bedtime?

➤ Does your child eat a large meal just before bedtime?

➤ Do you let your child eat chocolate or sweets or drink caffeinated drinks in the three hours before bedtime?

➤ Does your child have a bath before bedtime?

➤ Does your child skip bathtime regularly before bedtime?

➤ Is your child's bedroom too warm and/or too noisy?

➤ Is your child's mattress more than eight years old?

If you answered yes to two or more of the questions above, there are certain aspects of your child's lifestyle that are making it impossible for your child to get a good night's sleep.

Fortunately, there are many things you can do to make sure your sleep strategies for your child and their sleep are sound. The following guidelines will help.

➤ Establish a bedtime ritual for your child and make it consistent so that your child always goes to bed at the same time each night, even at weekends. Bear in mind the time that your child has to get up in the morning during the week and how many hours of sleep they need a night. Try and avoid your child having long lie-ins at weekends because it will make it harder for them to go to sleep at their normal bedtime that night and so their sleeping pattern will shift. Read Chapter Seven about the bedtime rituals. Following a consistent bedtime ritual is the key to solving many sleep problems.

➤ Review Chapter Four to see if physical problems may be the cause of your child's lack of healthy sleep.

➤ Taking the TV and computer out of your child's bedroom and limiting how much TV they watch can make a significant difference to the amount of sleep your child gets. If your child has a mobile phone, don't let them take it to bed with them. For more information on the bedroom environment and how sleep problems can be solved by making changes here, read Chapter Five.

➤ Making sure your child has a comfortable mattress, pillow and bed wear will help your child to sleep better. Look at the advice in Chapter Six.

➤ In Chapter Ten you will be given advice on food and diet to check that your child is eating the right things and at the right time to help them sleep at night.

EARLY RISERS AND LATE SLEEPERS (LARKS AND NIGHT OWLS)

The amount of sleep that we need is genetically determined. About 10–15 per cent of children have a biological tendency to wake up early in the morning. These early risers, popularly known as larks, are full of energy immediately, tend to be most alert around noon, and then tire early, needing to go to bed soon after supper. Owls, on the other hand, are the opposite of larks and find it difficult to get up in the morning, preferring later bedtimes. Their best time is late in the day and peak awareness is typically after 6 p.m. Children tend to become night owls in their teens because of a shift in the timing of their circadian clocks.

Despite the popular belief that 'early to bed, early to rise, makes a man healthy, wealthy and wise', there is no scientific evidence to prove that larks are better off than night owls. What matters is that children are getting the right amount of sleep, whenever that is, and that it is restorative good quality sleep.

ADVICE FOR LARKS

If you want your lark to sleep for longer in the mornings, you can try to put them to bed later by about 10–15 minutes each night until they are going to bed a whole hour later than normal. This may work, but many true larks will wake up early no matter what time you put them to bed. This may not matter to you if you are an early riser yourself (and as the tendency to be a lark is genetic, this may well be true!).

However, if you are not a natural lark and would like to be able to sleep in a bit, the best thing you can do is to persuade your child to stay in their bedroom until a reasonable time, even if they have woken up early. For children who are too young to be able to tell the time there are sleep training devices such as lamps that come on when they are allowed to get up and disturb mummy and daddy, or you can set an alarm clock and tell them they have to wait until they hear the alarm before coming out.

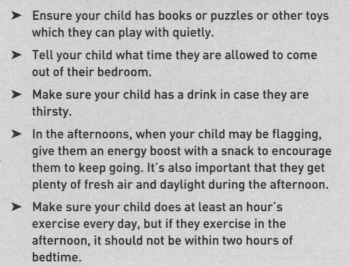

Tips For Dealing With Your Lark

➤ Ensure your child has books or puzzles or other toys which they can play with quietly.

➤ Tell your child what time they are allowed to come out of their bedroom.

➤ Make sure your child has a drink in case they are thirsty.

➤ In the afternoons, when your child may be flagging, give them an energy boost with a snack to encourage them to keep going. It's also important that they get plenty of fresh air and daylight during the afternoon.

➤ Make sure your child does at least an hour's exercise every day, but if they exercise in the afternoon, it should not be within two hours of bedtime.

Not all children who wake up early in the morning are genuine larks. Check that there aren't other reasons why your child is waking up early in the morning. Some examples might include:

Sunlight: is your child being woken up by light coming into their bedroom? If you find that your child only tends to wake up early in the summer months, then this is probably the case. Make sure you have thick curtains or blackout blinds that cover the windows properly so that no light can get in and wake your child.

Noise: for children with sensitive hearing, early morning noises can often be the cause of early waking. If there's an easy way to stop the noise, such as moving your child from a bedroom overlooking a noisy street to a room on other side of the house, then that's perfect. If this is not an option, then try setting the radio to white noise or to start playing at a low volume about half an hour before your child normally wakes up. This may drown out the sound of the harsh noises that wake your child.

TV: some children wake themselves up early to watch a particular TV programme. Make a rule about what time children are allowed to start watching TV in the morning. A favourite TV programme that is on too early can always be recorded for watching later.

ADVICE FOR NIGHT OWLS

Children who go to bed late cannot make up the hours of sleep they need by lying in in the morning when they've got school to get up for, so it's important your child goes to sleep at a reasonable time. If your child does not already have an established bedtime, make sure that they do.

Tips for Dealing With Your Night Owl

➤ If they are used to going to bed very late, start by bringing the bedtime earlier by 15 minutes and keep on moving it until it reaches the bedtime that gives them the amount of sleep they need.

➤ Help make bedtime a calm time, even if, for biological reasons, your child isn't able to go to sleep immediately. A relaxing bath and soothing music helps to create a feeling of sleepiness.

➤ Ban the TV and computer after a certain hour and suggest reading a book or other more calming activity.

➤ Wake your child at the same time each morning, even at weekends, so that they are more likely to be sleepy at night.

➤ Give your child a healthy, energy-giving breakfast to help them feel alert in the morning.

➤ Make sure your child gets enough exercise, but not too late in the day. The hour before bedtime should be reserved for winding down, not for strenuous activity.

HOW LONG SHOULD IT TAKE MY CHILD TO GO TO SLEEP?

The short answer is about 20 minutes, but this is very dependent on the individual child. Some children are perfectly happy to wind down in bed by themselves (see opposite). However, a recent study conducted by the University of Auckland in New Zealand found that children who had at least an hour's exercise a day fell asleep quicker than their sedentary peers. Those who didn't exercise took 26 minutes to fall asleep, while those who did took just 6 minutes.

And it doesn't mean that your child needs to spend a full continuous hour exercising; short bursts of activity are just as conducive to a good night's sleep. Once again we see just how important exercise is to a good night's sleep – and vice versa. Getting the balance right makes for a healthier, happier child.

MY CHILD TAKES TOO LONG TO GET TO SLEEP

There are parents who are not worried about how their child sleeps; what they *are* worried about is the length of time it takes for their children to fall asleep. Often they'll hear their child babbling, talking to themselves or playing with toys in their bed long after lights out.

We have been led to believe that if our child doesn't fall asleep immediately after being put to bed it's a bad thing. However, if your child doesn't show any distress, there is no need to worry. Your child is fine, and is probably one of those kids that takes a while to wind down before falling asleep. If your child is babbling, talking, singing or just rolling around on their own without calling out for you, it's likely they are giving you the message that they enjoy daydreaming and playing alone.

The thing to remember here is that every child is different. Some children want to be in their parents' company as much as they can, others need alone time. Some kids feel overwhelmed with constant interaction. And some kids have revved-up physiological systems that take a while to wind down. Sometimes that means they need your help with that calming-down phase (and you'll know that from their cries of distress), but sometimes they're doing fine all on their own, with no help needed from you.

> If your baby or toddler takes *for ever* to fall asleep, here's a few things you might want to consider.
>
> ➤ Once your child does fall asleep, do they sleep for a healthy period of time? If so, then there may not be a big problem for you to fix. If your child ends up sleeping

in later than you'd like, then consider an earlier bedtime so that they have time to wind down.

➤ If you and/or your partner are introverts, could it be that your child shares that trait and that the period before sleep is a time when your child gets those 'alone time' needs met?

➤ Are there too many distractions in your child's crib or bed that may be promoting more play and less sleep? If you have lots of toys, especially ones that buzz and blink and play music, then these things may be too stimulating when it's time for sleep. One or two stuffed toys, a blankie, soother or lovey are fine, and this sort of thing might just be enough to provide a soothing atmosphere.

I hope that what you have learned in this chapter has given you insight into your child's sleep patterns. As you know, not enough sleep leads to irritability, bad behaviour, poor concentration and problems with schoolwork, so make sure that your child gets between 9½ and 13 hours of sleep a night, depending on their age. While each child is different, I've provided you with guidelines on how much time your child should sleep at night as well as tips on how to deal with your lark or night owl.

Sleep is just as essential to a healthy lifestyle as good food and exercise, and should be made a priority. One of the more important points I hope you've taken away from this chapter is that consistency is vital to creating good sleep patterns in your child. Ensuring that your child goes to bed at the same time each night and gets up at the same time every morning, even at weekends and holidays, will not only set good sleep patterns in the short-term, it will help your child establish good sleep behaviours that will carry on into their adult life.

However, some children do experience more extreme sleep-related problems than the ones outlined here, which I'll tackle in the next chapter.

FOUR

Sleep Problems

Trouble sleeping is one of the most common problems experienced by toddlers and young children and most parents will know what it's like to have had difficult nights with their child. I certainly do, and I know that when your child has difficulty sleeping it affects your own sleep, leaving you exhausted and wanting to do anything you can to solve the sleep problem as quickly as possible. According to the National Sleep Foundation, more than two thirds of children aged under 10 experience some type of sleep problem which their parents think to be significant.

There are, of course, many different types of sleep problems – difficulty getting to sleep, waking in the night, nightmares and waking too early are just some of these – and there are many different causes of sleep problems. The good news is that most of these sleep problems can be solved quite simply without needing to resort to medical help. As a physiotherapist, I can provide practical and common-sense suggestions to prevent your child developing sleep problems. Hopefully my advice will ensure that your child, as well as everyone else in the family, will get a better night's sleep.

REFUSAL TO GO TO BED

From the age of about two, many children will try and put off going to bed and do anything they can to prevent bedtime. Stalling going to sleep and finding a variety of reasons to stay up – such as asking for just one more story, or another glass of water, crying or having a temper tantrum – can happen at naptime, bedtime or if a child wakes in the middle of the night, and it can make the whole experience of bedtime a miserable one which many parents dread. As a result of delaying going to sleep, these children often feel tired in the morning, are hard to wake up and irritable during the day.

If this is the case with your child, the first thing to do is to establish why your child is so determined not to go to bed. There could be a number of reasons and understanding what the reasons are is the key to solving the problem.

NOT TIRED

A child who is wide awake is not going to want to go to bed and trying to make them will often lead to bedtime battles. Check how much sleep your child is actually getting and when. If your child is having a long nap late in the afternoon then perhaps you are putting your child to bed too early or putting them down for a nap too late. Work out how much sleep your child needs for their age (see Chapter Two, pages 22–3) and try to adjust naptimes and bedtimes accordingly. Maybe your child no longer needs their daytime nap if they are getting enough sleep at night and it is time to drop it.

NOT ENOUGH EXERCISE DURING THE DAY

A recent study of 500 children showed that for every hour a

child is sitting – whether watching TV or reading a book – it took an extra three minutes for them to get to sleep. So making sure your child is physically active (though not too much in the hour before bedtime as they need to have a wind-down period) and not too sedentary will help them to feel tired and ready for bed.

As a physiotherapist I know the importance of exercise and keeping fit for our children (and for us as adults). Unfortunately, I have seen a growing number of children today becoming overweight through lack of exercise and eating unhealthily and this can often result in sleep problems, as well as putting children at risk of some serious medical conditions like heart disease and Type 2 diabetes; it also puts unnecessary stress on their growing bones. Every child should have 60 active minutes of exercise a day, but many children don't get this – partly because many parents don't know how much exercise their children should be getting. It shouldn't be difficult. An hour a day may sound like a lot but this doesn't have to be taken all in one go. If it's easier, you can divide the time into 15-minute slots throughout the day. And exercise will help your child feel tired at bedtime and sleep well throughout the night.

Tips and Tricks to Get Your Child Up and Running

➤ Walking to school and back home again is good exercise. If you live too far from school to walk all the way, try parking the car a few streets away and walking the last bit to school. You can make walks more fun by playing games like I Spy or spotting different types and colours of car so that children hardly notice they are exercising. Another good way to encourage children to enjoy walking is to give them a pedometer so they can see how many steps they have taken; this gives them a sense of achievement. Stopwatches are good too, so you can time how long it takes you and see if you can beat your time the next day. At weekends, you can encourage your child to enjoy walking by getting a map out and planning a route for a fun walk together.

➤ Tell children about the games you used to play at school in break time and teach them how to play them. Give your child a skipping rope to take to school, for example, or show them how to play hopscotch, which they can play with their friends.

➤ Do exercise as a family. Children love to do things with their parents and are much more likely to want to take part in physical activity rather than sitting in front of the TV if they can do something with you. Go to the local leisure centre and swim or skate together. Go for a family bike ride or try entering the family in an event like a fun run or bike ride.

➤ Tailor exercise to suit your child. If your child is not sporty but likes photography, take your child on a walk with a camera to see what interesting pictures you can take. Or perhaps your child likes cookery – so walk to the shops with your child to buy the ingredients.

➤ Take a Frisbee, kite or ball with you to play with when you go for trips to the park.

➤ If you have a garden, encourage your child to play outside as much as possible. Some children may like to help you with the garden, especially if you let them have a small patch to grow their own flowers or vegetables.

➤ In wet weather when you have to stay indoors, active games like hide and seek or even interactive sport video games can provide good exercise. Put some music on and get your children to dance around together.

➤ Praise your child for being active and, if more encouragement is needed, make a reward chart. Your child can stick a sticker on the chart every day they have completed a whole 60 minutes of being active.

EATING THE WRONG SORT OF FOODS

Eating healthily is just as important as doing enough exercise. As we'll see in Chapter Ten, certain foods eaten too close to bedtime will act as a stimulant keeping your child awake. Make sure your child is not eating a large meal too close to bedtime and check their diet. Regular meals and healthy snacks will help your child to sleep well and at the right time.

OVERTIRED

This may sound like a contradiction in terms but a child who is put to bed too late may get so tired that they become irritable, cranky and overtired, which makes going to sleep much harder. Try and keep to a consistent bedtime with a bedtime ritual that children look forward to and make sure that it is not too late for your child.

AFRAID OF THE DARK

Children with vivid imaginations or who are particularly sensitive may resist going to sleep because they are afraid of something. From the ages of four to six, children's imaginary and magical thinking starts to develop and this can lead to fears that there are monsters under the bed, and from the age of about seven children are able to understand the concept of cause and effect. This allows an even wider array of fears and worries to develop – an unexplained noise that could lead to some imagined disaster, for example. If this is the case it's important to be reassuring and sympathetic but also to be practical and think of ways to make the dark less frightening. Climb into your child's bed and try to see the room through their eyes. Perhaps allow a night light to stay on through the night or give your child a torch to keep by their bed. Playing soothing music can help, particularly if it masks the household sounds that cause the fear. Encourage your child to sleep with a comforter or soft toy that will give them security. Allowing them to come into your bed to be comforted by you and to co-sleep with you is an option that some parents may wish to take, although you may have difficulties in persuading your child to go back to their own bed again when you want them to.

> *Six-year-old Eden* couldn't go to sleep unless his mum was present and the lights were on. He said he was scared of the dark and of monsters, spiders and wasps. He had also started asking about dying and death.
>
> Eden had needed to have the light on to go to sleep since he was three, but the situation became worse after the Christmas holidays. It became clear that he was watching the same films and TV programmes as his older brothers. His mum realised that what he was watching had a powerful effect on Eden and had reinforced very normal fears that are common to all of us, such as fear of the dark, fear of dying and fear of animals such as spiders, snakes and monsters.
>
> To help Eden feel more secure when it was time to sleep, his mum ensured that his lights were left on dimly in his bedroom and bought him a 'special torch' which he kept close to his bed. The lights were left on in the hall and in the bathroom so that he could use the toilet without fear of darkness and shadows. She talked through Eden's fears with him and ensured that discussions before bedtime revolved around things that he enjoyed. Eden's mum also let him rearrange his

bedroom so that he was happy where everything was in his room. As part of his bedtime routine, Eden's mum made sure that before bed she read him pleasant 'happily ever after' stories, so that he had nice images in his mind before he went to sleep.

By playing down his fears gently but firmly and distracting him on to happier matters Eden soon moved on from this normal part of his childhood.

If you have established that there is no practical reason why your child is resisting bedtime, you know they're not hungry and they don't need another drink, then you need to be firm and consistent in the way you respond to your child's delaying tactics and set well-defined limits.

Tips for Setting Limits

➤ Have a consistent bedtime ritual that includes things your child looks forward to and enjoys – a bubble bath, story, etc. – and spend some time with your child. Sometimes children don't want to go to bed simply because they want to be with you, especially if you've been out at work and they haven't seen you much during the day.

➤ Even if it's the easy option, don't let them watch TV or play computer games just before bed instead of spending time with you. If you have given them quality time as part of the bedtime ritual, played with them, talked to them and listened to them, then that may help them accept bedtime more easily and it will make it easier for you to be firm about sticking to bedtime rules. You don't have to feel guilty about putting your child to bed.

➤ Explain that bedtime means bedtime and that your child must stay in bed after the lights have been turned out so that they know what is expected of them.

➤ Make sure that your child has had everything they need before you put them to bed – a drink or snack, trip to the loo, that they've got their favourite teddy and that they are tucked in, etc.

➤ Don't stay in the room until your child has fallen asleep but leave the room so that your child learns to fall asleep on their own – and they learn correct sleep associations.

➤ Make a reward chart and stick it up in your child's bedroom. For every night your child goes to bed without a fuss and stays in bed without getting out again, they can put a sticker on their chart.

GROWING PAINS AND OTHER ACHES AND PAINS

Nocturnal leg pains, also called 'growing pains' and sometimes despairingly called 'groaning pains', are very common in young children, with one in five children experiencing them at some stage especially during their primary school years.

Typically the pains are felt in the thigh or calf muscles and may be worse after a lot of physical exercise, although this is not always the case. They usually happen at night and, although they are harmless (no damage is happening to the bones or muscles), the pain can be enough to keep children awake. Boys and girls are equally affected and some children have growing pains on and off for many years until their mid-teens.

No one knows exactly why children have growing pains and there is no treatment for them. They do not affect how a child walks and runs and they don't make a child unwell so you don't need to see your doctor other than to establish that there is no more serious reason for the pains.

In my work as a physiotherapist, I see a fair amount of children with aches and pains. Sometimes they are associated with poor posture from sitting at the computer or playing with a hand-held console – make sure your children have chairs that they can pull in close to the table, and don't let them spend too long at the computer. Children generally start off life with good posture but over the years bad habits can creep in, especially because of the sedentary lifestyles that our children are leading. Encourage your child to stand properly – like a soldier or a ballerina, with their head up, shoulders back and tummy in. I always recommend sturdy rucksacks for carrying heavy schoolbooks, with heavy books packed first and lighter things on top. Other aches and pains often come from children overdoing it at sport. The bones grow faster than the muscles, which may be a source of some of the pain, and in order for the muscles to catch up, it may help to get some advice for stretching, strengthening and postural exercises for your child.

Children heal so much faster than adults if they injure themselves: a nasty bruise can disappear within a few days and a sprained ligament can get better within a week. If the problem persists do seek out the advice of your GP.

If growing or other pains are keeping your child awake at night you can try giving them painkillers, such as paracetamol, or a heat treatment such as a hot water bottle. Massaging the legs can also be soothing – if your child finds this too painful you should see your physiotherapist and/or doctor in case there is a more serious reason for the pains. Lots of hugs and reassurance from you that the pains won't last long and that they'll feel better in the morning will help too.

*During the summer holidays, nine-year-old **Oli** regularly woke his parents up in tears, complaining of aches and pains in his knees and thighs. This would happen at least two or three times a month. His parents would massage his thighs, use some heat on them and send him to bed. These pains were totally unconnected with physical activity. He had no other physical difficulties during the day.*

However, when the new school term started, Oli's knees were aching after indoor football. This persisted for four months, when his parents took him to the GP who reassured them that what Oli was experiencing was growing pains. Their doctor referred him for physiotherapy where he was taught stretching exercises for his thighs and calves as well as advice on posture. His physio reassured him that these aches and pains were a normal part of growing up and that the problem would soon stop. She also suggested shock-absorbing footwear to help alleviate some of the stress day-to-day life placed on his growing joints.

Within nine months Oli no longer had the growing pains but did experience the occasional ache at night which made him happy because he knew that he was going to be tall like his dad.

NIGHTMARES

You may remember having nightmares as a child – a really bad dream that woke you up because it was so frightening and which can stay vividly in your memory for years. Perhaps you still have them and know how scared they make you feel. Children usually first begin to experience nightmares from around the age of two, but they are most common in children between the ages of three and six years old. While some children may only have one or two in this time, other children can have them frequently, which can more seriously disrupt their sleep.

Although scientists are learning a lot more about dreams, both good and bad, it is not fully understood why children have nightmares, although it is thought that they are related to the normal anxiety and stress that are a part of growing children's lives as they process their memories of the day while they are asleep. Nightmares take place in the later part of the night during dream sleep.

There is not much you can do to prevent your child from having nightmares, apart from making sure your child hasn't been watching a scary or violent film before bedtime or been reading a frightening story. Instead you need to be able to comfort your child if they do have one. Give your child lots of reassuring hugs and talk to them quietly and in a soothing voice. Be calm and stay with your child for as long as they need you to, even if that means staying until they fall asleep again. Some children may be frightened of going back to sleep and the nightmare returning. Reassure your child that it is safe to go back to sleep. Talking about friendly monsters, like the ones in the film *Monsters, Inc.* who themselves are frightened of children, may help here, rather than just telling them that monsters aren't real. To your child, monsters *are* real.

Many children will remember their dream in the morning and want to talk about it. If they do, you can help by listening and making it less frightening by making up a happy ending to the dream. But some children may not remember their dream or not want to talk about it, in which case don't make them.

NIGHT TERRORS

About fifteen per cent of children have occasional night terrors, particularly between the ages of two and six, although they can occur at any age. They are not thought to be harmful and are considered quite normal but, even so, witnessing your child having a night terror can be extremely alarming and upsetting, especially the first time it happens. They occur early in the night, about 90 minutes into the sleep cycle when a child is in deep sleep, and can last anywhere between 5 and 30 minutes. When a child has a night terror, they will scream out loud, they may sit bolt upright and will look truly terrified with their eyes wide open but they will not see or recognise you and, amazingly, they will not wake up. In some cases, children may even get out of bed, they may be breathing fast and sweating but they are still asleep. When the night terror passes the child will go back to their passive sleep state and in the morning they will remember nothing about it.

Although it is horrible to see your child experiencing a night terror, it's important not to panic or to wake your child to try and comfort them. Remember, they are not aware of what's happening and, if you wake them and they see your panic and distress, that will makes things worse. There is nothing you can do while the night terror is happening except make sure that your child doesn't hurt themselves by thrashing about or falling out of bed or bumping into things if they start wandering around. There are, however, a few things you can do to minimise the occurrence of night terrors:

➤ Be sure your child gets enough sleep. The most common cause of night terrors is sleep deprivation, so check how many hours your child sleeps for and whether this is enough for their age.

➤ Make the bedtime ritual as calming and peaceful as possible (see Chapter Seven). If there are things going on in your child's life that might be upsetting or causing stress, try and talk to them about their worries.

➤ Review your child's diet and check that they are not eating things that could be disrupting their sleep. Allow your child to have a drink of hot milk with honey in it which is soothing and sleep inducing.

➤ Remember the importance of physical activity during the day. Healthy activity releases neurohormones, which relax both the body and the brain, especially at night.

BED-WETTING

Wetting the bed while asleep, also known as nocturnal enuresis, is very common in children especially under the age of about six or seven. About 50 per cent of all 3-year-olds and up to 40 per cent of 4-year-olds wet the bed several times a week and 20–25 per cent of 5-year-olds are not dry every night. As children get older, the problem decreases so that by the age of 10 only around 5 per cent of children wet the bed and then only occasionally. It is more common in boys than girls. There are various reasons your child may wet the bed:

➤ They may just be slow developers – and this may be hereditary. If you or your partner wet the bed as children there is a greater chance your child will.

➤ They may have a lower functional bladder capacity (the volume of urine a bladder can hold before starting to empty) than children who don't wet the bed.

➤ Some children sleep so deeply they simply aren't woken up by signals that tell them they need to go to the loo.

If your child drinks a lot before they go to bed, they may produce a lot of urine during the night that their bladder is unable to hold. Try not to let your child drink too much before they go to bed and make sure your child has been to the loo before bedtime. Take them to the bathroom again just before you go to bed – they won't properly wake up and will go straight back to sleep again afterwards.

If your child has previously been dry for a long period and then starts wetting the bed this may be a sign that your child is anxious or unsettled. You may find that your child starts to wet again if they are upset or coping with big changes in their life, such as when a new baby arrives in the family or when they start school. It may help if your child talks to a counsellor or trained mental health professional if the problem continues but usually, once the stress has passed, the bedwetting stops.

Remember that your child cannot help wetting the bed, and they are not being lazy or naughty. If you are patient the bedwetting will probably stop without any special treatment. However, if your child is over six and still wetting the bed at least once a week or if your child has been dry for a long period and then starts bed-wetting again and it persists, you may want to talk to your GP as there are various techniques you can try to help resolve the problem which, particularly in older children, can be upsetting or embarrassing. Some doctors may recommend medication, which can help but the treatment most commonly advised is a training technique called the 'bell and pad' or 'enuresis alarm'. This involves putting a pad underneath your child's sheet that is connected to an electric buzzer or bell. The alarm sounds when your child starts to wet the bed, waking your child up enough so that they can go to the bathroom. In time, your child will learn to wake up without the use of the alarm to go to the loo and so become dry at night. Reward charts are also recommended: reward your child a star for every dry night they have.

SNORING AND SLEEP APNOEA

It is estimated that about 25 per cent of children aged between 3 and 7 snore at least sometimes and about 12 per cent snore often. The noisy breathing of snoring results from the vibration of air going through the upper airway and it happens during sleep because this is when the muscles relax a bit making the airway a bit smaller. A number of things can cause snoring: coughs and colds, which lead to sinus congestions, and enlarged tonsils or adenoids that may block the airway; passive smoking can also cause children to snore as the smoke can cause the nose, throat and mouth to swell, making it hard to breathe.

In most cases the snoring is not a problem to the child

(though it may keep others awake who are sharing a room) and the children are healthy without any other symptoms. However, in about 3 per cent of children, loud snoring can be an indication of a more serious breathing problem called sleep apnoea.

Sleep apnoea is a term that means not breathing properly during sleep. There are many different types of sleep apnoea but the most common is called Obstructive Sleep Apnoea (OSA) and is caused by a physical obstruction of the upper airways by, for example, abnormally large tonsils and adenoids. Although the disorder is most common in overweight men and the risk of getting it increases with age, children do suffer from it and it can take a heavy toll on their sleep patterns. As a result of the airways being blocked the sleeper can stop breathing for up to 30 seconds before taking a noisy breath. Finally the child has to wake themselves up in order to catch their breath and go back to sleep although they may not remember waking up. This can happen up to 600 times a night. Naturally enough this leads to the child being very tired the next day and having difficulty with schoolwork and behaviour.

Children with sleep apnoea are also more likely to wet the bed, perhaps because the lack of restful sleep means they are less likely to wake up when their bladder is full. They also tend to get more nightmares and night terrors.

For children, the most common remedy is to remove the tonsils or adenoids which in 85–90 per cent of cases solves the problem. If your child snores loudly most nights, and wakes up tired in the morning often with a headache then you should arrange for your child to see the doctor.

SLEEPWALKING AND SLEEPTALKING

Both sleepwalking (somnambulism) and sleeptalking (somniloquism) are common in children and, though it can be unnerving for a parent to see their child walking or talking in their sleep, children who do it usually only do so occasionally and outgrow it by the time they reach their teens.

As many as 40 per cent of children aged between 3 and 7 may sleepwalk at some point or other. Sleepwalking can range from a child just sitting up in bed with their eyes open to walking aimlessly around the house or even wandering outside. Wherever they go while they are asleep, they won't remember any of it in the morning.

Sleepwalking usually occurs an hour or two after your child has gone to sleep during the deep sleep stage of their sleep cycle and when waking up is more difficult. It may last anywhere from a minute or two up to half an hour. While getting out of bed and walking around is the most obvious symptom, sleepwalkers may also sleeptalk but not respond when spoken to, and be clumsy. Although their eyes are open they are 'unseeing'. Bedwetting, sleep apnoea and night terrors may also accompany sleepwalking.

Sleepwalking can be triggered by lack of sleep, illness or stress, and eating the wrong foods near bedtime. As always, making sure your child gets enough sleep and has a good bedtime ritual is important and may help to prevent episodes of sleepwalking. Otherwise the most important thing you can do for a child who sleepwalks is to make sure they don't come to any harm. Don't let your child sleep on the top bunk of a bunk bed, put a stair gate up so they can't fall down the stairs, and keep all doors and windows safely secured. Don't try and wake your child, which might be difficult in any case and if you succeed could frighten or confuse them. Instead gently guide them back to bed.

Sleeptalking is even more common than sleepwalking and can happen in any stage of sleep. As with sleepwalking, your child probably won't remember it in the morning. Some children will just mumble and be unintelligible while others can speak quite clearly. If you talk to your child while they are sleeptalking they may not respond or, if they do, their response may not make much sense.

In most cases, sleeptalking is nothing to worry about and it will stop in time. Following the advice for healthy sleep in this book should help to prevent the activity sooner rather than later.

NARCOLEPSY

Narcolepsy is a rare chronic sleep disorder which results from the brain's inability to regulate sleep–wake cycles and which leads to excessive daytime sleepiness and cataplexy – a condition where you suddenly lose control of your muscles and collapse when you are angry, laughing or excited. Although it is more common in adults, children do suffer from it and because it is difficult to diagnose it is thought that there may be more children suffering from it than is realised. The four main symptoms of narcolepsy are:

➤ **Falling asleep at any time during the day.** This happens uncontrollably and can happen very suddenly at any time and any place such as at the dinner table or in the middle of a conversation, at a party or when they're sitting still. This is referred to as excessive daytime sleepiness.

➤ **Suddenly becoming floppy.** A narcoleptic child can suddenly become floppy at any time during the day as if they were asleep but when they're awake. A child will know what's going on around them but can't move. This is called cataplexy and can often be triggered by emotion – most commonly laughter.

➤ **Sleep paralysis.** When a child wakes up from sleep the brain wakes up but the body is paralysed and the child can't move or open their eyes.

➤ **Hallucinations.** Children with narcolepsy experience odd sounds or dream-like images upon awakening which they can remember and describe. These are called hypnagogic hallucinations.

Narcolepsy is a frightening condition for children which can have a damaging effect on their school and social life. A child with narcolepsy should be seen by a sleep specialist. Although there is no known cure, regularly scheduled naps can help and medication may be needed.

HYPERACTIVE CHILDREN

Sleep problems are very common among children who are hyperactive or who suffer from ADHD (Attention Deficit Hyperactivity Disorder), which is characterised by lack of concentration, a need for almost constant attention and restlessness, even when asleep. Research indicates that as many as 70–80 per cent of people with ADHD have difficulty sleeping, particularly in falling asleep – in one study, these children took up to 2 to 3 hours to fall asleep compared to less than 40 minutes for those without it. Additionally, many children with ADHD also suffer from sleep disorders such as sleep apnoea.

Helping children with ADHD to sleep better can have a significant effect on their behaviour, enabling them to focus and concentrate better at school, and calming them down. As well as putting into practice the general techniques for promoting sleep – yes, the bedtime ritual! – scientists also believe that sleeping pills can make a difference. In a study where children with ADHD were given sleeping pills containing dopamine there was a marked improvement in their sleep and an improvement in their level of attention, their hyperactivity and their sociability. Do always check with your doctor before giving your child sleeping pills.

Although a lot more research needs to be done into the links between sleep and hyperactivity, it would seem probable that making sure children get a healthy night's sleep can make a significant difference to their condition.

COUGHS, COLDS AND OTHER COMMON ILLNESSES AT BEDTIME

Once your child starts going to school, they are likely to start getting coughs and colds too – on average, preschoolers have six to eight colds and respiratory infections a year. It's a fact of school life, especially between October and April. Not surprisingly, the symptoms of these childhood illnesses – a runny or blocked-up nose, sneezing, watery eyes, sore throat and general achiness – which can last for up to two weeks, make it difficult for children to get to sleep, or can wake children up during the night.

Tips for Helping Your Child Get Over Coughs and Colds

➤ Give your child honey: forget the medicine! Doctors now think that the best remedy for soothing coughs and colds for children over a year old is buckwheat honey or other dark honey. (It's important not to give honey to a child under one because of the risk of botulism, a type of food poisoning.) Drug companies now agree that cough and cold medicines should not be given to children under four, and that buckwheat honey can be more effective. It has the added bonus that most children like the taste. Half a teaspoon for children aged between two and five, and a whole teaspoon of honey for children between six and eleven, given half an hour before bedtime is all that is needed.

➤ Give your child plenty of fluids: coughs and colds can be very dehydrating so drinking a lot is important. It will also help to loosen the mucus.

➤ Avoid foods that increase mucus, such as dairy, soy and orange juice.

➤ Use saline nasal drops: non-medicated saline nasal drops will help clear a blocked nose and make it easier for your child to breathe at night.

➤ Keep air moist in the bedroom: use a cold mist humidifier to help soothe irritated nasal passages.

➤ Elevate your child's head: raise the mattress at the pillow end of your child's bed by putting some large cushions underneath to relieve sinus pressure and help breathing.

➤ If your child is over four and you think they need over-the-counter medication, check with the pharmacist or doctor that they are appropriate and safe for their age and condition, and ask if there is anything in them which may prevent sleep, such as caffeine.

➤ Most importantly, if your child has any illness they will need extra amounts of hugs and loving care. Your love and attention is the best remedy for helping them recover quickly and settle back into healthy sleep patterns.

STRESS AND SLEEP

We'd like to think of our children's lives as being blissfully carefree and without anxiety or a worry in the world. But the reality is that many children suffer from stress and do have worries, or are sensitive to the stress of others around them. Even very young children can suffer from stress and research has shown that stressed children are more likely to have sleep problems than children who aren't stressed.

There are many situations that can potentially cause a child to be stressed. Very young children from the age of around one can experience stress if they are separated from their mother. The stress is increased at naptime and bedtime when a child realises that you are leaving them alone to sleep and they may often cling to you and cry. This is a stress that children will naturally outgrow as they learn that when you leave the room you haven't gone for ever and will be back, but it's important to do what you can to minimise the stress in the meantime and to help your child to sleep well without anxiety. Encouraging your child to adopt a comforting toy to take to bed with them may help, as well as explaining calmly that you will be there in the morning when they wake up. Practising with short separations during the day will help teach your child that you will come back.

In toddlers and preschool children, research has shown that pushing them to learn too much too quickly can cause stress which may result in tantrums, bed-wetting and nightmares. Parents may think they are helping their children to become high achievers but in fact the opposite may be true if the children's stress levels result in sleeping problems.

For older children, there can be even more reasons for feeling stressed. Schoolwork, homework, sporting and social pressures can pile stress on to children who can end up unable to sleep at night because of their worries.

Problems in the family can be a major cause of stress in children and research has shown that, in families where the parents are fighting frequently and are hostile to each other, children lose sleep over it. The negative effects of the sleep loss, which disrupts attention and increases irritability and poor behaviour, can be long lasting. Other stresses within the family, such as money worries, are keenly felt by children who, if they are sensitive, will often feel a huge burden of worry on their shoulders.

Whether your child experiences stress will of course depend a lot on your child's temperament. A sensitive, anxious child is less likely to be able to deal with stress than a child who has a more laid-back nature. Temperament plays a very important part in a child's ability to sleep well. Researchers have found that children who are described by their parents as temperamentally difficult, intense, needy and fussy babies have more sleep disturbances and sleep problems than children with easier natures and this can persist into later years. These children will need a more sensitive approach to their sleep problems.

Knowing your child's personality and being aware of what might be stressful for them in their lives is vitally important so that you can help relieve their anxiety.

> ### If You Think There is Potential for your Child to be Stressed:
>
> ➤ Talk to your child and be a good listener. Give them as many opportunities as possible to share their problems with you.
>
> ➤ Help your child to manage potentially stressful situations. If homework seems to be getting on top of your child, help them write an organised work plan and so on.
>
> ➤ If you are having marital difficulties then it's important to be aware of the impact on your children. Consider seeing a family counsellor to help your children understand and come to terms with what is happening.
>
> ➤ Keep healthy, consistent bedtimes in place.
>
> ➤ Try and create a relaxing and peaceful bedtime ritual to help soothe your child and de-stress them.

Children don't come with a manual and, if you think that your child may be suffering from any of the above, take your child to your local doctor who will be able to guide you in the right direction for further help.

Finding out what kind of sleeper your child is, dispelling any anxieties your child may have surrounding getting to sleep and dealing with any sleep problems will take you a long way on your journey to getting a good night's sleep for your child. Back this up with ensuring your child's sleeping environment is as comforting and inviting as possible and you will find that your child will go to sleep more readily and easily than before.

FIVE

The Bedroom

Is your child's bedroom helping or hindering a good night's sleep? It may sound obvious but the room your child sleeps in can make a huge difference to how well they sleep. If your child feels comfortable and happy in their bedroom they are more likely to sleep well. Equally, an uncomfortable room that has negative associations for your child will make it more difficult for your child to sleep well and can contribute to nightmares or other night-time fears and anxieties, such as monsters under the bed. Your child spends more time in their bedroom than in any other room in the house so it is highly important that it should be a place where they feel relaxed and calm, which reflects their personality and which they look forward to going to sleep in.

For many children, their bedroom is more than just a place to sleep; it is also their playroom, their study and their living room. Times have certainly changed. The bedroom is now a place of overstimulation with computer games, social networking, electronic toys, games consoles, information gathering, TV watching, texting, playing, homework, and often two or three of these activities may be taking place at the same time. While it is important for your child to spend leisure time in their bedroom, this must be balanced with the fact that too much cerebral stimulation combined with too little physical activity makes going to sleep difficult. Sleep should be the primary function of the bedroom so, whether your child is doing their homework or playing with their toys in the bedroom, the atmosphere should be kept tranquil and restful, helping your child to unwind so that when bedtime comes they are in the right mood for sleep.

SLEEPING ENVIRONMENT

A well-designed bedroom is not necessarily one that has all the latest fashions and high-tech gadgets, but is one that provides the best sleeping environment for your child. This should be a space that feels comfortable, safe and secure and where your child is happy to go to bed at night. There are many things you need to consider when designing your child's bedroom and it's often helpful to get your child involved in these decisions. What we parents think our children may like and would prefer them to play with, such as nostalgic wooden toys which look nice on the shelf, may not necessarily be what our children want, such as colourful, plastic toys. Although you will need to set some boundaries (some children may have imaginative ideas that are beyond your budget or desires!), by discussing the design of the bedroom with your child as well as thinking about the practical considerations you are more likely to end up with a room that your child will sleep well in.

What to Think About When Designing Your Child's Room

➤ How dark is your child's room?

➤ How noisy is your child's room?

➤ How warm is it?

➤ Does your child have a TV, mobile phone or computer in the bedroom? If so, what are the rules surrounding the use of them?

➤ How old is your child's bed? Does it sometimes double up as a trampoline?

➤ Is your child sharing with a disruptive sibling?

➤ What sort of pillow are they sleeping on?

➤ What sort of bedding are they using?

➤ How is their room in the dark? Are there any disturbing shadows?

As your child gets older, the look and feel of their bedroom will evolve and change to reflect their personalities. The bedroom of a preschool child will be very different from that of a 10-year-old who increasingly wants to assert their independence. But whatever the age of your child, you need to remember that their bedroom should be conducive to good sleep. If your child is not sleeping well, now would be a good time to have a look at your child's room and consider the following things.

Colour and Decoration

Forget blue for boys and pink for girls. There is a wide range of ideas, colours and colour combinations that may be more suitable for you and your child. Tailoring the room to suit your child's needs and how he uses the room is important. For example, you could divide the room into zones for different activities with different colours.

It is well-known that colours have a strong influence on our mood and feelings even if we don't realise it. Blues and purples can be calming for an overactive child but can also be cold. Reds and other strong colours, though warm, can be overstimulating. Pinks, however, will soothe and calm. Bright walls, in particular brilliant white, can reflect so much light even at night that it prevents sleep. Greens, on the other hand are thought to have a balancing and harmonious effect, which is one of the reasons you feel calm after a long country walk. Think about the colour of your child's room and how it makes you feel and the effect it might have on your child. The ideal colours for a bedroom are pale shades of pink and green: the pink will send your child off to sleep and the green will help your child feel refreshed in the morning.

Similarly, posters and other wall decorations need to be thought about. Are there any images on the walls that might be frightening, overstimulating or subconsciously causing anxiety? While some children may be happy to have pictures of fighting soldiers or knights or something scary from a favourite TV programme adorning their walls or their bedcovers, these images may prevent more sensitive children from sleeping well. Have a look at the decorations and ornaments in your child's room and see if there's anything there that might contribute to sleep problems and discuss it with your child.

Harry, aged nine, loved football. Not only was he a great fan of watching the game (he never missed a Liverpool game, ever) but he was also a great player, scoring for both his school team and for the local club. The teams did well and they often won trophies that Harry proudly displayed on a table at the end of his bed. The only problem Harry had was that it took him ages to get to sleep and he would wake up frequently in the night. After a lot of time and thought and discussion with Harry, his parents finally made the connection between the football trophies and Harry's sleep problems. Although Harry's trophies made him feel proud, they also made him feel anxious about whether he would be able to continue to play well and win again. They were the last thing he looked at before the light went out and his brain was unable to relax and unwind ready for sleep. Once the trophies were moved to different place, however, Harry was able to think about more relaxing things which not only helped him to fall asleep more quickly but also stopped his night-time awakenings.

Bedroom Accessories

Children love to play pretend and 'grown ups' and it's nice to provide them with things with which to recreate the adult world. Furniture stores have come a long way and you do not need to spend much money in order to fill your child's room with great things to play with. A cool set of table and chairs could be the setting for a teddy bears' dinner party as well as somewhere for your child to get creative with crayons and paint. Funky boxes look great and can be used for all kinds of imaginative play, as well as providing storage for toys once it's time to pack up. And creating a comfy cushion zone gives you and your child a special space for storytime.

Lighting

Children – and adults – sleep better when it's dark. This is because it's darkness – or the absence of light – that triggers the release of melatonin in our bodies, which is the hormone that makes us feel sleepy. When it is light, our bodies stop producing the hormone so we stop feeling sleepy. Bearing this in mind, it makes sense to be able to keep your child's room as dark as possible when you want them to sleep, particularly in the summer months when the long light evenings can make it difficult for children to get to sleep, and the bright mornings wake your child up prematurely. Here are some suggestions for keeping your child's room as dark as possible:

➤ Take a look at the window coverings you have and see how much light they let in. Insulated curtains that have a durable foam back lining will keep the light out on the summer days and absorb more light and heat during the winter months. They will help to keep the room cool in the summer and warm in the winter.

➤ Blackout material to line existing curtains or to make blinds is also very effective at blocking out the light and can make a real difference to the length of time your child sleeps. As a temporary measure you can use dustbin liners to cover windows. If you have blinds that do not adequately cover the windows and there is a gap on either side, stick some tape down the sides to block the light. Window shutters are also effective at keeping out the light.

➤ Doorways may let in light, either natural or artificial, under the door, so try and keep these covered. Door snakes are useful here, or other draught excluders. Think about the way the door hangs in relation to the source of the light and perhaps consider changing the way it hangs.

➤ A canopy that fits over your child's bed is a fun way of providing darkness and is especially useful if you don't want to darken the whole room that siblings may be sharing. Canopies are easily portable so are also ideal for travel and can be used to ensure less light in hotel rooms or when staying away from home.

➤ Other lights, apart from natural light, that can prevent your child from sleeping well include LCD lights from electrical items, particularly if they blink or flash on and off and your child can see them from the bed. The light from a TV or computer can have an effect on melatonin production and consequently affect your child's sleep at night. Even the lights of a digital clock placed near your child, can wake them when they're in a period of light sleep. Also ensure light-reflecting objects, such as mirrors, are not directed at your child.

➤ In general, lighting should be soft in the bedroom, and if you can fit a dimmer switch to lower the lighting at bedtime, this is very useful.

If your child is afraid of the dark, you will need to make allowances. While it is still a good idea to make sure all sources of natural light can be excluded, there are plenty of lighting appliances that allow you to control your child's exposure to light. There has been much research into the effect of keeping a light on at night and, although the ideal way to sleep is in darkness, if your child is frightened of the dark, providing a night light which is kept on throughout the night can be comforting and reassuring and help your child to sleep.

Light at Night

➤ Plug-in light sockets that automatically come on when it gets dark and fade when it gets light. If your child is worried about waking up in the night and not being able to see to go to the bathroom, use a plug-in light socket in the hallway which will give visibility but minimises light exposure.

➤ Moonlight lamps give off a calming green tone rather than a yellow sunlight tone and are more conducive to restful sleep.

➤ Glow-in-the-dark stickers for the ceiling

➤ A bedside torch

➤ Hang up a string of chain lights to give off a comforting glow throughout the night but which don't heat up

➤ Make sure that any night lights are positioned so that they give off a glow rather than shine directly into the eyes

Temperature

As yet, sleep experts have not agreed on an ideal temperature for a good night's sleep – it seems to vary a little from person to person. But, in general, sleep research indicates that most people, including children, sleep better in a cooler room. Our internal body clock controls our body temperature and this has an effect on when we feel sleepy and when we feel awake. At night, our body temperature drops and this, combined with the lack of light, triggers our melatonin production, which makes us feel sleepy. Our body temperature is lowest at about four in the morning, after which our temperature begins to rise and we start to prepare for waking up.

So how cool is cool? Obviously you don't want your child to be too cold, just as you don't want them to be tossing and turning because they're too hot. Depending on how many covers your child has on their bed, you should be aiming for somewhere between 16–18 degrees Celsius (62–65 degrees Fahrenheit). Fans or air-conditioning may help in the summer. Make sure that fans are moving the air around in the room but are not directed at your child. Air-conditioning is best used to cool a room before your child goes to sleep and then turned off at night. Clean the vents regularly and have the unit professionally cleaned and checked at least once a year.

Many parents also believe in the health benefits of keeping the window open to allow fresh, cool night air to come in providing it doesn't let too much noise in at the same time. How fresh the night air is will, of course, depend on where you live but the quality of the air in a child's bedroom is certainly worth paying attention to, especially if your child suffers from asthma or other allergies. An ideal night-time humidity level is 60–70 per cent. A humidifier (which will release moisture into the room to help ease breathing), a dehumidifier (which takes moisture out of the air) or an air purifier can help to create the best air quality and promote better sleep.

Noise

Children's sensitivity to noise varies greatly from child to child. Some children can sleep through anything; as a boy my grandfather once slept through the noise of an air-raid siren going off without waking up at all. On the other end of the scale there are children who can be woken by the slightest sound.

In general, toddlers tend not to be as distracted by noise as adults. Apart from the first 10–15 minutes after your toddler has gone to sleep when they are still in the light stages of sleep, you don't need to creep around the house trying not to make a sound because relative silence makes your child more sensitive to noise. As children get older, however, they tend to become more sensitive to noise and will sleep better in a quiet room. Like most of us, children will be woken up by sudden loud noises.

Achieving a quiet environment can be difficult, particularly if you live in a large household or noisy neighbourhood. Try the following suggestions:

➤ Work out if the noises that disturb your child are coming from inside or outside the house. Squeaking floorboards, noisy pipes or radiators, etc. may need attention.

➤ If the noises are coming from a busy road outside or noisy neighbours and it's practical, you could consider moving your child to the back of your house away from the sound.

➤ Thick, insulated curtains will help to deaden sound as well as black out a room.

➤ Children may also find it easier to go to sleep with a low background noise, or white noise, which helps to drown out sounds from elsewhere in or outside the house. White noise is produced by a combination of different sound frequencies that masks out other sounds. A good example is the hum of a fan or air-conditioner, or the sound made by a vacuum cleaner or washing machine which is strangely soothing. Don't worry, I am not suggesting that you clean your house all night long to help your child get to sleep and stay asleep! There are plenty of CDs of white noise available to buy, or you can buy a white noise machine. A cheaper alternative is to make a recording of your washing machine to play to your child before they go to sleep, and even keep it on all night long.

➤ Similarly, tapes of lullabies and other soothing music can help your child to sleep.

➤ Interestingly, the sudden absence of noise can also wake some children (as you may have observed on long car journeys when your sleeping child wakes the instant the engine is turned off) and children who are used to going to sleep with background noise may find it harder to settle when they stay somewhere quiet and without noise.

Smell

A clean fresh-smelling bedroom is a much nicer environment for your child to sleep in than a bedroom that is full of strong odours. There are two areas to think about. First, there are the smells that may be contained in your child's bedroom itself. Rotting food, dirty socks or wet towels hidden under the bed are common causes of nasty smells, as is any collection of dirty laundry. Other culprits include animal cages and fish tanks, which can quickly smell nasty if not regularly cleaned out, particularly in the hot summer months. Opening windows to let fresh air in every day helps, as does a quick spray of air freshener, providing it is not too strong. Adding a few drops of lavender or chamomile oil, which is especially good for children, to your child's pillow can create not just a fragrant-smelling room, but aid sleep too.

Secondly, you should consider how smells from other parts of the house may drift into your child's bedroom. Cooking smells from the kitchen, however delicious, may keep your child awake if they are feeling hungry. You could consider investing in an extractor fan or hood for your cooker if you don't already have one. Other smells, like wood smoke, can affect children with asthma or other allergies and should be avoided, as should tobacco smoke. Ask visitors or anyone who smokes to smoke outside.

TVs, mobile phones and computers in the bedroom

Does your child have a TV or computer in their bedroom? If so, they are one of the 79 per cent of children (or 4 out of every 5) aged between 5 and 16 who do, according to market research agency ChildWise. Their research shows that 63 per cent of children lie in bed watching the screen and two-thirds of children, particularly the youngest, watch television before they go to school. On average, British children now spend 5 hours and 20 minutes in front of a screen every day.

So having a television and computer in a child's bedroom is obviously popular, but is it a good thing? In terms of how well your child sleeps, research certainly suggests that it is not. Studies show that children who watch TV in their rooms get less sleep. Research conducted at the University of Haifa examined 444 middle school pupils aged 14 who were asked about their sleep habits and use of computers and television. It found that children with TVs in their room went to sleep half an hour later than those without a TV while waking up at the same time in the morning, effectively losing 30 minutes of sleep a night. Some children will also get up earlier in the morning to watch TV at the expense of sleep. As we've seen in Chapters One and Two even 30 minutes' less sleep can have a major impact. While this is only a relatively small study of children a bit older than the ones we're looking at in this book, there are many other reasons to think carefully about allowing a TV in your child's bedroom:

- It is much more difficult to be in control of what your child watches on TV if they are doing it in their own bedroom. You may not be aware of a programme they have watched that scares or frightens your child, giving them nightmares and a fear of the dark and going to sleep. Younger children, in particular, may not be able to make the distinction between what they see on TV and real life, so it can be especially confusing and/or disturbing.

- While it is possible to restrict what your child looks at on the computer, it is harder to do so with television.

- It is also harder to be in control of exactly how much your child watches TV and when they are watching it. Some children will stay up late, past their normal bedtime to watch a TV show they like, or wake up early to do so. The temptation is always there, even if they know they are not meant to do it, and this can be disturbing too.

- Watching TV before bedtime can cause inappropriate sleep associations. Children who become used to watching TV at bedtime may find it difficult to get to sleep without it. At the same time, the stimulation children get from watching TV or surfing the net on their computer before bedtime can make it harder for them to wind down, relax and mentally switch off to allow themselves to get to sleep easily.

- There appears to be a connection between too much TV watching and obesity. Instead of doing more active things, TV encourages a very sedentary lifestyle, which makes burning off calories more difficult. In turn, obesity can lead to sleep problems such as sleep apnoea, snoring and breathing difficulties while asleep.
- Watching TV at bedtime is often at the expense of a bedtime book. Reading your child a book at bedtime not only helps to develop your child's sense of language, but is also a shared experience which is comforting and reassuring for children, making it a gentle transition from wakefulness to sleep.

Mobile phones are similarly popular and an increasing reason why children are losing out on sleep. More than half of British children aged between five and nine own a mobile phone and this figure looks set to rise as a range of kiddie-phones with simplified buttons designed for children as young as four are set to hit the market. Aside from the health concerns surrounding the use of mobile phones, the findings of a new survey reveal that 40 per cent of children with mobiles phones are sleep-deprived on school nights as they stay up to text their friends. The advice of sleep experts is that no child should be allowed a phone until the age of 12 and certainly not in the bedroom.

Sleepy Gadgets

You may be amazed at how many toys and gadgets there are on the market that are designed to help make bedtime more fun and sleep easier whether at home or travelling. From the traditional hot water bottle in fun animal covers and soft toys that you put in the microwave to warm up the bed and be a huggable comfort, to teddies that breathe or sing your child to sleep. Other gadgets with a more obviously practical use include humidifiers, which add moisture to dry air to make breathing easier at night, monitors that allow you not only to hear your child but to see them too while they are asleep, and sleep-training clocks and lamps which are timed to go off/come on in the morning to tell your child when they are allowed to get out of bed.

All these toys and gadgets have passed safety standard tests (check the labels for a sign of this) and if they do help your child to get to sleep or to sleep better and for longer, then that is wonderful. It might be worth borrowing from a friend first to see if a toy/gadget works before going out to buy a more expensive item.

SHARING WITH SIBLINGS

Do you have children who share a bedroom and do they both sleep well? Sharing a bedroom with a sibling may be something your children choose to do because it makes them feel happier and more comfortable, or it maybe something they have to do because of lack of space. There is nothing wrong with sharing a room. Children can quite easily share bedrooms and sleep very well, especially if the children are close in age. Similar sleeping patterns and shared interests make sharing a room companionable and often the healthy sleep of the older child can encourage good sleeping habits in the younger child.

Problems may arise, however, if one child has a sleep problem or a problem with their health that disturbs the other. If this is the case, and both children are getting a disrupted night as a result, you will probably have to separate them until the sleep problem has been resolved. Once the problem sleeper has learned how to sleep well, the sibling can then return to the shared room.

As children get older, the need for their own independent space often becomes greater and it's important to listen to them and check how they are feeling about sharing.

SAFETY IN THE BEDROOM

How safe is your child's bedroom? This question is not just directed at parents of preschool children – although there are particular considerations for this age group – it's important that bedrooms should be as safe as possible for children of any age. Consideration should be given to electric cables, which should be kept tidily to the edge of the room and out of the way so children don't fall over them, and all electrical outlets should be covered. Even quite old children who are naturally curious may try and stick their fingers into the holes of plug sockets to see what happens unless these are covered up.

Have a look at the furniture in your child's room and make sure that any tall items such as wardrobes and book-shelves are fixed securely so that they can't topple over. If favourite objects are placed too high up on a shelf the temptation to climb up to get them may be too great and be a potential hazard. Be careful, too, about glass in a child's bedroom. You may want to consider replacing glass picture frames or any other glass coverings with plastic ones to prevent broken glass in your child's room.

Make sure that you have a working smoke detector and, if you have gas appliances, a carbon monoxide detector in or near your child's bedroom. Once a month check the batteries are working and change them at least once a year.

BEDROOM AS A SAFE HAVEN

You may be satisfied that your child's bedroom is as safe as you can possibly make it, but your child needs to feel safe and secure in it too. A child's bedroom is their sanctuary and should be a place they can relax in, a cosy nest, where peaceful thoughts help them to sleep happily and well. Try and have a look at your child's room through their eyes. Get into their bed and see the view they have – you may be surprised. My son started sleeping only on one side and in one area of his bed after I put a storage unit in his room. I climbed into his bed in the dark to try to see if I could learn anything. I felt as if the world was closing in on me. I have since rearranged his furniture so that he can see around the room clearly with no cupboards in the way and he is now sleeping in all of his bed.

Sometimes a room can feel too big to be restful, or too cluttered with too much going on in it. If your child's bedroom is also their playroom and their study room, they may be prevented from going to sleep easily by seeing the mass of unfinished homework still to do, or the unfinished game still to be played. If this is the case, see if you can divide the room into different areas for their different activities using screens or furniture. Think how you can make the area where they go to sleep as separate from their normal daytime activities as possible and free from anything that might cause worry or anxiety. A nice thing to do, which helps give your child a sense of security as well as a connection to the family, is to put familiar objects – such as family photos – around the room. And try not to create negative associations with the bedroom by using it as a place to send your child to as a punishment. Your child is far more likely to sleep well and healthily all night long if they think of their bedroom as a happy place and look forward to going to bed.

Once you have done everything you can to provide the best sleeping environment for your child, it is time to look at the bed itself to make sure that it too is both comforting and comfortable.

SIX

The Bed, Pillow and Bedclothes

For the first two years of their lives, children spend more time in bed than anywhere else. After that, children are still spending roughly half their life in bed. So providing them with a really good-quality bed and mattress and comfortable bedclothes is vitally important to ensure their growing bodies get the support they need, as well as giving them the most comfortable night's sleep. Getting the right bed for your child is one of the most important purchases you can make. But it can be difficult to know where to start. There are so many different types and designs of bed available, and the choice of mattresses, pillows, duvet covers, etc. can be overwhelming. What sort of bed should you buy? What is the best mattress? When should you move a child from their cot into a big bed?

The answers will vary according to your child and to the size and design of the bedroom. Some children are ready to move into a big bed months earlier than other children. Some children will sleep better in small beds and others find big beds more suitable. You will need to take your child's personality and preferences into account. At the same time there are certain general guidelines you should follow which will help you find the best bed and bedding for your child to give them a really good night's sleep.

TIME FOR A BIG BED

Moving from a crib or cot into a proper bed is one of the milestones in your child's life – and in yours too, as it is a sign that your child is growing up and leaving babyhood behind. From a practical point of view it can make a difference to your life, at least for a while, as your child discovers the freedom of being able to get out of bed whenever they want, no longer confined by the safe and secure bars of their cot. The trick, of course, is to find a bed they want to stay in.

So when is the right time to you move your child into a bed? The most generally accepted advice is to move them when your child starts to climb out of their cot, making it no longer safe, or once they've reached 89 centimetres in height (35 inches). The other most common time for moving a child out of their cot is when there's a new baby on the way. For most children this is anywhere between the ages of eighteen months and three and a half years old.

Whatever the reason, and whenever you decide to do it, you want to make the transition as easy as possible. Spending some time thinking about the type of your bed your child will feel most comfortable and secure in, where to put the bed and what to put on the bed are all details that will help to make the move as easy as possible to ensure the best sleep.

WHAT TO CONSIDER WHEN BUYING YOUR CHILD'S BED

Safety
This *is* the most important factor to consider. The bed needs to be strong and sturdy and all the screws and joints need to be secure – double-check this if you've assembled the bed

yourself! Make sure there are no sharp edges or points. Choose a bed that is low to the ground so that your child won't hurt themselves if they fall out of bed. You may want to buy safety rails that can be detached once your child has adjusted to sleeping in a bed. It's also a good idea to put something soft around the bed such as a soft rug or quilt in case your child does fall out of bed. Modern beds should have passed safety tests. If, however, you are buying a second-hand bed or using an old family bed, then buy a lead paint test kit (available from most hardware shops) and check that there is no lead-based paint on it, which is poisonous.

While we're on the subject of safety and beds, a word of caution about children using beds as trampolines! It is of course very tempting for children to bounce on the bed, but this can be dangerous. Not only do children risk bumping their heads if they bounce too high or hurting themselves if they fall off, but there is also a risk of children injuring themselves from broken wires inside worn-out mattresses. Although not common, some older mattresses are constructed with wire to hold the mattress coils in place, which have caused nasty injuries to children bouncing on them. If you have an older, cheap mattress the advice not to jump on the bed is particularly important.

Design

When looking at the promotion of children's beds, you would be forgiven for thinking that the way a bed looks and its fun factor are the two most important criteria for buying one. They aren't, or shouldn't be; however, you will want to choose a bed that appeals to your child and fits in with the overall design of their bedroom. For the really young end of the market there are novelty beds where the bed is designed in the shape of a car, digger, train, jeep, pirate ship, fairy bower, etc. For older children, too, there is a wide choice of style.

Location

Certainly to begin with, it is a good idea to put the bed in the same place as the crib was. Your child is used to getting to sleep in that place and to that view of the room when it's night-time. If one side of the bed is against the wall, you need to make sure that your child cannot become trapped between the side of the bed and the wall.

CHOOSING THE RIGHT TYPE OF BED

When it comes to choosing the bed you want, you have a lot of choices, not least of all size. Recent statistics show that many parents are now choosing full-sized or double beds for their children to allow greater freedom of movement while sleeping (we turn about 20–40 times a night) as well as to make it more comfortable for both parent and child when sharing bedtime stories and quiet talks. It also means that the bed will be big enough for your child for some years to come. However, you will need to consider how much space there is in the bedroom. You don't want the bed to take up all the space so there is no room for your child to move about in the room. The following table lists standard bed sizes, but it is a general guideline only as bed sizes are not always standard and may vary depending on country of origin.

Toddler:	70 x 145 cm
Single:	90 x 190 cm (3 ft x 6 ft 3in)
Double:	135 x 190 cm (4ft 6 in x 6 ft 3 in)
King:	150 x 200 cm (5ft x 6 ft 6 in)

Toddler Bed

These are smaller and lower to the ground than a full-sized single bed and with built-in safety rails and head- and tailboards. They are a good transition between the cot and a big bed, still cosy in size and providing safety, and easy to get in and out of. Many of them are made to appeal directly to toddlers with clever designs of cars or castles on them and this can be a great way of encouraging small children to want to sleep in a bed. The disadvantage is that your child will soon outgrow a toddler bed – most of them are designed for children from eighteen months to five or six years old – so you will need to buy a bigger bed in a few years' time.

Regular Beds

If you decide to move your child straight into a regular-sized bed, you have the choice of buying a bedstead made out of metal or wood and separate mattress, or a divan bed which consists of a base for a mattress and has no headboard. The divan base usually incorporates drawers so that they are a good choice if you are tight on space. You can buy a removable bed side while your child gets used to his new bed.

Bunk Beds/Cabin Beds

Bunk beds and cabin beds (whether high sleepers or mid-sleepers) that utilise the space underneath the bed with a desk, or play area – are only suitable for children from the age of six for safety reasons. For the six-plus age group these beds are not only great fun, but can be enormously useful as space-saving devices. The important thing, always, is to consider the safety angle. High beds should have high bed rails so your child can't fall out. Make sure, too, that the ladder is easy to climb up and down and that your child uses the ladder and doesn't try and jump from the top bunk.

CHOOSING THE RIGHT MATTRESS

Even if your child is not like the princess in the fairy tale of the princess and the pea, choosing the right mattress for your child can make the difference between a good night's sleep and a bad one. Fortunately these days you won't need to pile mattresses on top of each other to provide ultimate comfort! But even if your child is not a sensitive 'princess' and can seemingly sleep happily wherever and on whatever they are put, it is worth buying the best mattress you can to make sure your child's body is getting the proper support. As a physiotherapist, I know that this can help avoid back problems and other pains in later life. For this reason, I really would recommend buying a new mattress and not using a second-hand mattress for your child to sleep on. It's worth remembering, too, how close your child's face is to the mattress while they are sleeping. It's estimated that adults sweat as much as half to a full pint of fluid a night, so old mattresses are really not hygienic. The general advice is that we should change our mattresses every eight years.

Mattresses can be made from all sorts of different materials and constructed in different ways. You can choose from basic sprung mattresses, pocket sprung mattresses, foam ones, coil mattresses, air mattresses, latex and hypoallergenic mattresses. Eco-friendly parents might consider buying an organic mattress made of completely natural materials such as coir fibre, cotton and wool. These also dissipate heat and perspiration better. However, what is important is the level of support the mattress gives your child. Ideally you want a mattress that gives firm support without being uncomfortable.

You should never allow your child to sleep on a very soft surface such as a water bed, large beanbag, a foam pad or a feather bed for fear of suffocation.

Modern mattresses should all be fire retardant, but do check the label, especially if you are using a second-hand mattress.

Mattress protectors

To get the best use out of whichever mattress you decide to buy, and to make the mattress as comfortable as possible, it's sensible to buy a mattress protector too. A single mattress contains several kilograms of droppings from dust mites, microscopic bugs that live in mattresses, and every movement you make in bed sends a cloud of droppings in to the air ready to breathe in, which can be particularly difficult for asthma sufferers (please see below for more about allergies and asthma). A mattress protector or cover will prevent you or your child from breathing this in. Depending on the manufacturer, mattress protection can be described as mattress protectors, mattress covers, allergy bedsheets, allergy bed cover, anti-allergy protectors, anti-allergy bedding or allergenic bedding but all serve a very similar purpose. These are also available in a large variety of materials from synthetic materials such as polyester, vinyl and latex rubber, to more natural cotton and wool. Make sure that you buy a washable cover, though a water-resistant surface, while useful for protecting the mattress from bed-wetting, may not be as comfortable.

LOOKING AFTER YOUR MATTRESS

A new mattress should be aired for at least four hours to freshen and remove any aroma from storage before using. The mattress should be aired on a weekly basis by turning back the bedlinen for a few hours. Some mattresses, such as sprung mattresses, need to be turned every two weeks to keep their shape and avoid dips and an uneven sleeping surface. These mattresses, should have strong handles on the side to make turning easier. Other mattresses such as latex and foam mattresses do not need turning, but should be rotated lengthways about once a month to maximise their life.

In addition to using a mattress cover, cleaning the mattress with a vacuum will help to remove some of the dust mites that invariably live in any mattress, together with the dead skin that is lost at night. This is particularly important if your child suffers from any allergies or asthma, but is good hygiene for any child. You could also consider getting a mattress doctor to give all the mattresses in your house a professional clean once or twice a year.

PILLOWS

In my experience as a physiotherapist, a good pillow is just as important as a good bed for getting a good night's sleep. A pillow too big or bulky can cause poor posture in growing children, and an uncomfortable pillow will cause children to toss and turn and sleep badly. The right pillow, however, will not only give necessary support for your child's neck and spine and help prevent round shoulders but also make a wonderful comforter and many children will become very attached to their pillows once they get used to sleeping with one.

The main aim of the pillow is to preserve good posture. Posture is something that we normally think about with regard to sitting and standing but it also must be addressed in lying. If your child is on a very big pillow he will be flexed too far forwards or if he spends hours twisted to one side to watch the TV he could be setting himself up for neck and back problems in later life. The main aim is to keep the body in the mid-line position, which means that you are maintaining the natural curves of the spine to minimise stresses and strains.

As a physiotherapist I have seen an increase in children with neck and back pain over the past 20 years, which is obviously very concerning, and poor sleeping posture could be one of the contributing factors.

Most children will only sleep with a pillow when they move from their cot to a bed, usually at two to three years – it is not safe for children under eighteen months to sleep with one. Even then pillows are not essential, but children usually want to have one to be like everyone else; most of us sleep more comfortably with a pillow. Another reason to purchase a pillow for your toddler who is over two years of age is that many young children tend to get ear infections as a result of colds, and may also get a blocked nose; using a pillow to prop your toddler up at night will help ease the pain and allow him to breathe more easily.

Young children should start with a flattish and fairly firm pillow, though soft enough to be comfortable. Adult pillows are far too big and will not give your child the proper support. If you're not sure what kind of pillow will suit your child best, consider how they sleep. If your child sleeps on their back, a medium-firm pillow is recommended, while a firm pillow, supporting the neck, is best if your child sleeps on their side. A slightly softer pillow for cushioning and comfort is better for children who sleep on their tummies. You should avoid the very soft goose down or feather pillows. If you do choose feather pillows for older children over the age of five or six, check the pillows regularly to make sure that the feathers are not escaping as they can be a choking hazard.

> ### Broken Pillow Test
>
> To test the support of down and feather pillows, lay the fluffed pillow on a flat, hard surface. Fold the pillow in half and squeeze out the air. Release the pillow: one with support will unfold and return to its original shape; a broken pillow will remain folded.

For children who are asthma sufferers or who have allergies, choose a pillow made of hypoallergenic material such as latex foam, which provides very firm support and does not collect house dust, and avoid feather pillows.

BEDLINEN

When buying bedlinen for your child's bed you want to keep in mind what will be most comfortable for your child. Sheets made of natural materials such as cotton or linen, though more expensive than synthetic polyester, will provide more comfort. They are long-lasting, absorbent and suitable for any climate. Linen sheets give the most fresh feel for a bed, being light and cool. The disadvantage, apart from the cost, is that they are difficult to iron. Making sure that sheets are smooth and not crumpled when making the bed is important in helping your child have a more comfortable night's sleep. Fitted bedsheets are useful in this respect, but note that, because mattress sizes with the same names may vary, you must check that the fitted sheet size will fit the mattress. Check the measurements carefully before purchasing a fitted sheet.

The decision whether to use blankets or duvets as bedcovers is a purely personal one. For babies, you should always use blankets because you can layer them to get the right amount of warmth for your child – add a blanket or two in winter and use fewer in summer. Tucking your baby's blankets in makes them feel secure too. This is true, too, for children and it can be wonderfully comforting for them to be tucked in at night. But nowadays most children have duvets on their beds. The ease of making the bed together with the appealing range of designs for duvet covers make them the most popular choice.

DUVETS

The weight, softness and warmth of a duvet depend on its tog rating and filling. Tog ratings are based on a duvet's ability to trap warm air. The higher the tog rating, the warmer the duvet. As children are smaller than adults it means that their duvet traps more air and increases the level of warmth. Unless your child's bedroom is very cold, it is best to stick with a lighter weight duvet between 4.5 and 9 tog. If necessary, you can always use a blanket on top of the duvet in winter.

Duvets with natural fillings are soft, light and comfortable, in the same way that natural fibres help your skin 'breathe' more effectively. They are also highly resilient and tend to last longer than those with synthetic fillings. However, synthetic duvets are a practical choice if your child is allergic to feathers and down or if the duvet is likely to need frequent washing – natural-filled duvets should be professionally laundered.

BLANKETS

Soft woollen blankets make a very good bed covering for children. With blankets it is easier to get the level of comfort and warmth and bed temperature exactly right which, in children more than adults, may vary from one day to the next. The act of being tucked into bed at night can also be part of the bedtime ritual, which signals it is time for sleep. Even if children have a duvet as their main covering, a child can still have a blanket, throw or fleece blanket on top that can be tucked in over the duvet.

Many children also take a comfort blanket to bed with them and find that being able to stroke it and hug it and snuggle it makes them feel secure and helps them to sleep. There is nothing wrong with this, except for the times when the comfort blanket disappears and can't be found in time for bedtime. If at all possible, it's very useful to have an identical spare one in reserve, which may just work. Some children as old as seven or eight still have them, only finally outgrowing them when embarrassment with friends overcomes the desire for comfort.

Wool

Wool, though expensive, is an excellent fabric and particularly suitable for bedcovers. It is lightweight but because of its heat-regulating qualities will keep you warm in cold weather and cool in hot weather. It is water repellent, useful for spills and also for wicking moisture away from your body, which helps keep the body at a more even temperature. This can help you and your child get a better night's rest and sleep for longer. It is a natural flame retardant, having a low burning rate so it doesn't need to be treated with chemicals, and it doesn't get dirty easily. Washable wool fabric makes it easier to care for too so there is no longer any need to dry-clean woollen blankets.

SLEEPING BAGS

For children under the age of four, you can buy indoor sleeping bags, which are useful to prevent your child from kicking the sheets off and may stop your child from getting out of bed and going wandering. These are usually 2.5 tog and can be used all year round, apart from in the height of summer, and you can add or remove blankets depending on the temperature. You can also find 1.5 tog versions, which are suitable for summer and daytime naps. Under 1 tog is suitable for summer in hot countries. You can ensure that the child remains at the right temperature by adding or removing blankets.

You can buy inside sleeping bags for older children too. These are not intended to replace duvets or blankets as bed coverings, and should be used on an occasional basis when friends come over for sleepovers, or to snuggle in while watching TV. They can provide a comfortable night's sleep and their fun designs encourage children to think of bedtime as an enjoyable time.

If you are choosing an outdoor sleeping bag for your child, the amount of warmth it provides is the most important thing to consider. Sleeping bags come in two basic shapes. Mummy bags are usually better for children as they fit more snugly and have a hood that can be pulled tight around their head creating a lot of warmth and insulation, but the rectangular shape will suit children who tend to sleep with their arms and legs sprawled out. Again, sleeping bags are not intended to replace normal bedding for older toddlers and children, but they are a fun way to make sleepovers feel just that little bit more special.

BEDWEAR

While your child is still young enough to let you choose what they wear in bed, it's worth bearing a few things in mind. The first thing is comfort. When it's hot, your child will need something cool to sleep in like some lightweight pyjamas and, in the winter when it's colder, you will need warmer night clothes for them. Look at any buttons or other fastening which might be uncomfortable to sleep in, or frills on nightdresses such as lace around the neckline which can rub and cause irritation.

Secondly, you need to think about safety considerations, and in particular the risk of fire. Night garments need to be made of flame-retardant materials and should be fitted, not snug. Fitted pyjamas are better than billowing nighties, which can more easily catch fire. Obviously the pyjamas need to be loose enough to allow freedom of movement, but not too loose-fitting as to pose a risk.

As your child gets older, what they wear in bed will become a matter of personal choice. Some girls will prefer to sleep in nighties and others in pyjamas, while some boys will prefer short pyjama sets and others to sleep in long pyjamas. It's important to let your child choose what they feel most comfortable sleeping in to provide a good night's sleep. Some children feel so comfortable in their pyjamas that they would happily stay in them all day! However, it is best to discourage this. Having clothes that are worn only for sleeping in, not just helps to keep them clean, but also helps to reinforce the sleep cues – I'm in my pyjamas, so it must be time to sleep.

TEDDIES AND TOYS IN BED

A soft toy such as a teddy can often act as a comfort object that soothes your child when you're not there. This can be particularly helpful at bedtime when your child is going to sleep or if your child wakes in the middle of the night. Hugging the toy and feeling the soft fur against their cheek or lips is reassuring and may be enough to help a child get to sleep without needing you to be there too.

Children tend to receive a lot of soft toys when they are babies but there is usually one that particularly appeals to them more than the others and becomes the special one that is taken everywhere – and may remain a favourite for many years to come. If you do have any say over which toy your child chooses, try and encourage a toy that is not too big. You will need to make sure that they don't choose a toy that contains anything that could be either uncomfortable for sleeping with or potentially dangerous, in particular anything that could come off – plastic noses or button eyes are a good example.

Apart from the chosen comfort object, it is better if children don't take other toys to bed with them. My three-year-old son would love to take all his trains and cars to bed with him, but not only are metal objects in bed not conducive to a good night's sleep, a cluttered bed full of toys doesn't help good sleep either. We have a rule that he says good night to his toys before he gets into bed and just takes his one bedtime teddy to sleep with him.

ASTHMA, ALLERGIES AND DUST MITES

There is another reason for not allowing your child to take too many soft toys to bed – they are a wonderful home for dust mites. Dust mites are microscopic bugs that live in household dust and are a very common trigger for allergies and asthma. Their diet consists mainly of shed human skin so they particularly like to live in mattresses and bedding where they can find a plentiful supply, as well as in rugs and upholstered furniture.

Over 5.1 million people in the UK have asthma, a chronic disease in which sufferers have repeated attacks of difficulty in breathing and coughing. The number of children with asthma is very high: 50 per cent of all asthma sufferers are children. Allergies are also very common and children who suffer from either allergies or asthma often suffer from disturbed sleep. Not only do the symptoms of both conditions – breathing problems, coughs, inflamed nasal passages and itchy eyes – make sleep difficult but the body's immunological response to allergens disrupts systems set up to regulate sleep.

Although there is currently no known cure for asthma, 85 per cent of people are allergic to the dust mite excrement and dust mite skeletons found in every mattress, even if it's only a few months old. Reducing dust mites in your child's bedroom and making sure the bedroom environment is as clean as possible can make a significant difference to a child's symptoms and how well they sleep.

Jonny, six, was recently diagnosed with asthma, which accounted for his night-time coughing fits and the difficulty he had breathing after vigorous physical exercise. He was prescribed two inhalers, one was preventative and one was only to be used in a case of emergency. However, Jonny's mum soon learned that there were many more ways of protecting Jonny from possible asthma triggers and irritants, and the first place to start was the bedroom. As well as keeping the room exceptionally clean, vacuuming often and dusting shelves every day, Jonny's mum used air purifiers, which helped remove contaminants from the air. Another precaution taken was to buy mattress covers that provided an extra barrier for dust mites and other allergens. The great thing about the covers is that they took up no more space than a folded sheet would, so Jonny's mum took them with her to hotels and on sleepovers so Jonny had the protection all the time. Similarly she bought pillow covers, which served a similar purpose. Although the inhalers and medicine were vital to keeping Jonny safe and well, managing his surroundings was fundamental in keeping the asthma at bay.

Ways to Reduce Dust Mites and Other Allergens:

➤ Wash your child's soft toys frequently in hot water and then dry them in the tumble-dryer on the highest setting. Do check the washing instructions first to make sure toys can withstand high temperatures – you don't want to shrink your child's favourite teddy! You can also put soft toys in a plastic bag and put them in the freezer overnight as dust mites cannot survive freezing temperatures for more than five hours.

➤ Wash all of your child's bedding in hot water (at 54.4 degrees Celsius or 130 degrees Fahrenheit) and then dry it on a high setting in the tumble-dryer every few weeks. Hanging sheets and other bedlinen on a washing line collects pollens and moulds which can cause allergic reactions.

➤ Vacuum your child's bedroom at least once a week and clean the furniture with a damp cloth. Vacuum the curtains and your child's mattress too – it may not remove many dust mites but it will remove the dust they feed on.

➤ To avoid dust, try and keep your child's room as clutter-free as possible. If you can, keep most of your child's books and toys in a playroom or somewhere other than the bedroom.

➤ Take up the carpets in your child's bedroom. Carpets harbour dust mites and pollen, so a bare wooden floor will reduce them in the bedroom. Rugs that can be regularly washed can soften the effects of bare floors.

➤ Use allergy-proof mattress and pillow covers to prevent dust mites interfering with sleep.

➤ Reduce humidity in the bedroom. Dust mites love moist areas so a dehumidifier to keep humidity below 50 per cent will discourage them.

BEDBUGS

Another pest that can affect your and your child's health is the bedbug. Although seemingly eradicated in the UK in the 1980s, the bedbug is enjoying a resurgence in recent years. No one is quite certain why, although the boom in travel over the past decade may be one factor: bedbugs are very efficient and good travellers and can hitch a ride in your luggage. Once established, they are very difficult to get rid of. Contrary to popular opinion, bedbugs don't prefer unsanitary homes to clean ones.

Bedbugs are nocturnal and quite small – less than five millimetres (0.2 inches) in length. They are pale brown in colour, though that changes to a reddish brown after they've ingested your blood.

If you are infested, be assured that bedbugs do not

transmit any diseases but their bite often leaves a hard, whitish swelling. You will probably notice small spots of blood on the sheets, and you may also notice small black spots on bed joints or in the seams of mattresses – these black spots are its faeces. If you've been infested particularly badly you may notice an oily smell – this is created by the bugs' 'stink glands'.

Bedbugs are notoriously difficult to get rid of and if you've been infected it's best to hire an exterminator to make sure the job is done properly.

Getting Rid of Bedbugs

➤ Hire an exterminator, do not attempt to get rid of the bedbugs yourself by using insecticides

➤ Don't move the furniture out of the infected room as it can spread the infestation to the rest of the house

➤ Do not move out of the bedroom – bedbugs will go looking for warm bodies if none is available

➤ Change bedding two times per week and wash sheets in hot water

➤ Dry bedding in the tumble-dryer

➤ Use tea-tree oil

➤ Use a steam cleaner

➤ Use an electric blanket, but don't sleep with it on

Once you have made sure that your child has the best environment to sleep in and the most comfortable bed to sleep on, there are no practical reasons why your child should not have a good night's sleep. The next step to take is to look at your child's bedtime ritual.

SEVEN

The Bedtime Routine and the Daily Nap

To my mind, establishing a regular bedtime ritual, or routine, where you prepare your child for bed in the same way and at the same time each night, is the most important thing you can do to help your child get a healthy, good night's sleep. Allowing their children to choose how and when they go to bed depending on how they feel every night may sound like a great idea to those parents who dislike the notion of schedules in general, perhaps fearing they restrict freedom and creativity. Some parents may also find it easier in the short-term to wait for their children to fall asleep on the sofa before putting them to bed. But the reality is that children who lack a consistent bedtime ritual have more problems sleeping, are more sleep-deprived than children with one, and less secure. Going to bed at the same time and in the same way each night does not have to be complicated, and establishing good habits is easy; if you are consistent you will see that it can really improve your child's sleep.

You should also look at the way you sleep. Do you have a set time for bed or do you only get ready for sleep once your eyelids feel heavy? Children between the ages of three and ten are like a sponge, soaking up ideas and habits, and no role model is more important than you, their parents. Studies have shown that sporty children come from sporty families, and in my work as a physiotherapist I've noticed how children react to pain in the same way that their parents do. So, to ensure that your child has a healthy bedtime ritual, it's imperative that you should set an example by having a good one of your own. You'll be surprised at just how much difference it makes to your day-to-day life!

So why is a bedtime ritual so important? The American journal *Sleep* recently published the findings of a study in which 405 mothers of young children with mild sleep behaviour problems were shown how to follow a very simple bedtime ritual. This included a bathtime followed by a massage and then storytime before lights out. The results showed the routine had many benefits:

➤ It significantly improved sleep and bedtime behaviour in infants and toddlers – including the time it took for the child to get to sleep, the number of times they woke up during the night and how long they slept for.

➤ Toddlers were less likely to call out for their parents or get out of bed in the night.

➤ The reduction in the children's sleep problems meant that the mood of the mothers who were surveyed was considerably improved. This in turn had a beneficial effect on the children's sleep. Because the mother was less stressed, the bedtime experience for the child became happier, and this helped them fall asleep more easily too.

The Importance of a Bedtime Ritual

➤ It tells your child to expect sleep and helps them to unwind to prepare for it. An energetic child who has been doing active things all day needs to have a built-in peaceful time before bedtime to make the transition to a calm state so that they are ready to fall asleep.

➤ Schedules help children feel secure and safe because they know what is coming next; in fact, they thrive on it. If bathtime always comes after dinner and is followed by stories, they know that what happens next is sleep and are less likely to resist it.

➤ Research shows that a systematic approach to daily life leads to less stressful environments for young children. The familiarity of the bedtime ritual, the predictability and the clear boundaries you set will provide security for your child, which will help to calm your child and prepare them to feel restful before sleep.

➤ Instituting a bedtime ritual will improve sleep in your Infant and toddler and will also set them up for better sleep throughout their life. It's also been proven that a bedtime ritual provides a significant reduction in problematic sleep behaviours. And there's an added benefit for parents too, who find that their mood improves when their child gets a better night's sleep.

➤ A consistent bedtime ritual where you have set your child's bedtime, rather than your child deciding when they go to bed, puts you in control. Especially once your child starts school and has to be up in the morning by a certain time, it's important to know that they have been to sleep early enough the night before to get the sleep they need. Having a consistent schedule for going to bed means that you can be certain that your child is getting the amount of sleep they need. Without a set bedtime ritual, it becomes much more difficult to know when your child is going to feel sleepy and want to go to bed. This in turn makes it harder to schedule other activities and to organise your time and that of your child.

> ➤ It helps you to make sure that all the things that need to be done before bedtime, like having a bath and brushing teeth, are done in a coordinated manner, and, once these good habits are established, you no longer have to think about them.
>
> ➤ A bedtime ritual requires a commitment from you, which tells your child that their sleep is important to you. A good bedtime ritual will allow you to enjoy spending time with your child and make the end of every day an enjoyable experience for both of you.

Ben, age five, had recently stopped settling at his usual bedtime of 7.45 p.m. He used to be a great sleeper who had always slept through from 7.45 p.m. until 6.30 a.m., but lately he was struggling to get off to sleep.

His dad had started a new job which was more stressful and much further away which meant that Ben's dad was getting home an hour later than his former return time of 6.30 p.m.

When Dad came home he used to play 'rough and tumble' with Ben, but because he returned home later it meant that Ben's bedtime ritual was being delayed and Ben was getting excited just at the time that he was meant to be settling down. He started falling asleep in front of the TV and in the car, and was more irritable and cranky during the day.

Ben's mum implemented a strict bedtime ritual which involved quiet time, bathtime followed by night clothes and straight into bed with a story and reward chart every night without Dad getting involved initially. Ben was allowed to be the first one to wake

Dad up for rough and tumble early the next at and Dad put Ben to bed at the weekends.

Within two weeks Ben settled and his dad chose to work late two nights a week so that he could get back in time for Ben's bedtime ritual the other nights.

THE BEDTIME RITUAL

Every child and every family is different and there is no set of rules that has to be followed to the letter, but here are some suggestions. You will need to decide what works best for your family and for your child, and what is realistic for you to achieve. Think about what things your child enjoys and, depending on the age of your child, involve them in working out a series of steps for going to bed – for example, whether they prefer a bath or a shower, what toy they like to take to bed and which stories they like to hear. Work out the things that have to be included such as brushing teeth and putting on night clothes and then add the things that will make it enjoyable yet calming.

Once you have made these decisions stick to them. Being consistent is the key to making the new bedtime ritual work. Kids learn by testing boundaries and, when they see they can't get away with breaking the rules and no amount of trying will change the ritual, they begin to understand that there are set activities for the night and that bedtime is when they go to sleep. For this reason it's best not to make the new set of habits too complicated or over long. You will need to do the same thing every night and you don't want to shoot yourself in the foot.

Ideally, the bedtime ritual should be centred on the child's bedroom and the bathroom – coming downstairs or into another area of the house where there might be something interesting going on will easily distract your child and turn their attention away from sleep. Try not to rush the routine even if you are longing to get your child into bed and asleep so you can put your feet up. In fact, it may have the opposite effect: a child who knows you are rushing them may take longer to go to sleep, calling out for you after you've turned the light out to get more time with you. Also, if you try and rush the routine, you won't be allowing enough time for it to be enjoyable and it will become a chore that has to be done before bed rather than a time to look forward to sharing together. As a guideline, from getting out of the bath to lights out typically takes half an hour.

Include everything in the bedtime ritual that your child needs to do before going to bed so there is no excuse for them to get out of bed after the light has been turned out. So make sure that:

➤ they've been to the loo
➤ they've had a bedtime snack if they're likely to get hungry
➤ they've had a drink of water, or that a glass of water is beside their bed

If you haven't tried setting a bedtime ritual before, it may take a few days for your child to adjust but I would think that by the end of the first week your child should have accepted it – it's amazing how quickly children respond to new systems. Once your child has understood that there is a pattern to their bedtime, which you mean to enforce, they will stop fussing about being made to go to bed. There will be an end to bedtime battles and your child should fall happily asleep within 10–15 minutes of you leaving their bedroom.

A Typical Bedtime Ritual

Yours may include some or all of the following – you may even have other things you'd like to include:

> a relaxing wind-down period of low-key activities with a 10-minute warning before going up to bed
> a bath or shower before changing into pyjamas or night dress
> bedtime snack
> brushing teeth
> bedtime story
> a massage or quiet music
> prayers/bedtime poem
> hug and good night kiss

IMPLEMENTING THE RITUAL

Firstly, you need to decide when you want your child's bedtime to be. Work out how many hours sleep your child needs according to their age (Chapter Two, see pages 22–3), then work backwards from the time they need to get up in the morning. Then work out what things you will include in the bedtime ritual and estimate how long each thing will take to see what time you need to start.

The Wind Down

Before bedtime, your child needs to wind down and have a quiet time. How much time is up to you, but anywhere between 30 minutes and an hour. Quiet time is a chance to play, think and slow down. Here are some tips:

➤ Create a specific area or quiet zone.

➤ Decide which toys are acceptable for winding down and avoid noisy, exciting toys. You will know what quiet things your child enjoys doing most – reading, playing a game with you, doing a puzzle or listening to music.

➤ Avoid your child doing physical exercise in quiet time. While exercise throughout the day is, of course, important to help your child feel tired at bedtime, the increase in adrenalin has a stimulating effect, which makes it difficult for them to fall asleep easily.

➤ Avoid TV watching. Although 77 per cent of parents use TV as a pre-bedtime ritual and many parents allow children to have TVs in their bedrooms, it has been shown that watching TV before bed makes it more difficult for children to fall asleep and leads to less restful sleep. Children who fall asleep watching TV seem to have the most sleep disorders, with nightmares caused by TV programmes being a common problem. There is also concern that children are trading sleep for TV (see Chapter Five, page 80 for more about TV and the effect on sleep). However, if you do decide to allow your child to watch the television then check carefully what programmes are on and whether they are suitable for your child and for bedtime.

➤ Decide how long quiet time will last and five or ten minutes before it's time for your child to go upstairs to get ready for bed, give them a warning. This gives them enough time to finish what they're doing and be ready to go to bed.

➤ Make sure you and your child keep to the rules of quiet time.

Bath or shower

Having a bath or a shower can be a lovely way to relax at the end of the day and a great way to help prepare children for sleep. A warm bath calms a restless mind. It also sends the blood away from the brain to the skin surface and makes children feel relaxed and drowsy. As well as this, your child's body temperature, which has been raised by the warm water, will drop as soon as your child enters their cooler bedroom and this initiates a feeling of sleepiness. It also releases melatonin and, as the melatonin level rises, it causes the blood vessels to constrict which concentrates the blood around the vital organs causing the body temperature to reduce. It's important to make the water not too hot, though, as this will keep your child's body temperature too high, making them feel hot and uncomfortable. Adding bath oils or bubble bath scented with the essence of flowers such as lavender and chamomile that are thought to be particularly conducive to sleep is also helpful.

But while some children find baths relaxing, others may not. Some children find that bathtime wakes them up and makes them feel more alert. For younger children, there is the possibility of tears at being made to get out of the bath, which leads to stress rather than relaxation. If this is the case, it's better to schedule the bath or shower for the morning or before tea.

Bedtime story

I would highly recommend that you include reading a bedtime story in your child's bedtime ritual, and not just for little children. You may wish to do this in bed or in the comfy zone of the bedroom. Children as old as 12 or 13 still enjoy being read to by their parents, or additionally/alternatively listening to an audiobook. Not only does a bedtime story mean that children are staying still while they listen to the story and relaxing, but it can be a very enjoyable, bonding experience that you share as well as helping your child's literacy skills. How long you spend reading depends on how old your child is and how tired they are. You may need to set a limit if your child is always asking for just one more book/chapter/page/ paragraph! But this is where story tapes can be useful. After you have read for long enough, you can turn off the light and allow them to fall asleep listening to a story being read by someone else. Make sure the story is not too exciting or scary, as this may keep your child awake for too long.

Often children, especially preschool children, have a favourite story they want to hear over and over again. The predictability of it is comforting and soothing and, while it may be less exciting for you, don't think you can skip a line or two – your child will know and remind you that you've missed a bit. The important thing here is to enjoy the time you are sharing with your child. Children that get read to are also more likely to become readers, as it becomes a habit that is familiar to them.

Music

Going to sleep listening to soothing music can help many children unwind and fall asleep more easily. There is a wide range of music available designed to be listened to at bedtime which include lullabies, simple classical music and gentle repetitive songs. You could also try recordings of natural sounds such as bird song or whale song but be careful not to use the sound of running water too much because it may make your child want to go to the toilet. The advantage of listening to music is that it can mask the sound of other noises in the house that might be disruptive. If they are old enough, the child can also turn the music on themselves if they wake up in the middle of the night and need help to get back to sleep again.

Massage/Relaxation

Touch is the first sense to develop in humans and massaging your child gently as they lie in bed can be a very bonding experience which relaxes, soothes and comforts your child just before they drop off to sleep. Although stress is thought to be an adult problem, as I outlined in Chapter Four, children can suffer from stress too and this is a common cause of sleep problems. A massage can literally rub the stress away and make sleeping easier. It doesn't need to be particularly complicated. With very young children, a gentle stroking over the body is enough. As your child gets older, the massage can become more sophisticated to include different strokes applied to the feet, fingers and toes. Massage classes for parents are very popular and you should be able to find one in your local area. Alternatively, books can explain the different techniques and methods. Experiment a bit and see what your child likes. There are some good bedtime massage gels on the market formulated to help calm and relax too.

Prayers/Bedtime poems

You might use these as vocal cues to let your child know that it's bedtime. It might be something simple like 'Night, night, sleep tight, don't let the bedbugs bite' (though I never found this particularly reassuring!) or 'Love you, see you in the morning', which tells your child that it's time to go to sleep. It is something you say as you switch the lights out and leave the room.

Traditionally many children said a prayer before they went to sleep at night. Saying a prayer, or a bedtime poem if you are not of a religious persuasion, can be very comforting for a child especially if it is something you do together, and if it is done every night, will become a cue for sleep. You may want to make up your own prayer with your child. Alternatively you may want to repeat the words of traditional prayers which will soon become familiar to your child and will be learned by heart so they can say it to themselves when they need that comfort.

A BROKEN SCHEDULE

As with all routines, there are always going to be times when you can't stick to them or when the routine changes. It's important to be flexible – to recognise when your child has outgrown their routine and to make necessary changes such as a later bedtime, as well as to be prepared for when the routine can't be adhered to. Some children will find it harder to adapt to a broken routine than others depending on their temperament. But most experts agree that it can be a good thing for children to learn how to cope when the routine is broken as it teaches them how to be flexible as well as demonstrating that the world won't come to an end if the routine does change.

TIME CHANGE

Every year in spring and autumn, the clock changes and we gain or lose an hour. It takes most of us a little time to get used to the change in time, and we find it harder to get to sleep or wake up in the morning. Studies actually show that for two days after we 'spring forwards' and lose an hour's sleep, there's an average increase of up to 10 per cent of traffic accidents, more than at any other time of year. For children, the loss of an hour's sleep leads to less concentration too, as discussed in Chapter One, as well as moody and irritable behaviour so it's important to do as much as you can to prepare your child for the time change.

Time Change Tips

➤ When the clocks change in the spring, we lose an hour's sleep, so start putting your child to bed a little bit earlier a few days before the clocks actually change. You could begin on Thursday night going to bed 15 minutes earlier, then increasing it by 15 minutes each night until Sunday night when your child goes to be a whole hour earlier. Doing it in small stages may make it easier. Reverse the process when the clocks go forward, in the autumn.

➤ Use the power of light to help reset your child's body clock. Keep the lights dim by drawing the curtains for an hour before you put them to bed and use bright lights to wake them up in the morning. If possible, have breakfast outside in the natural sunlight or in a room that has a lot of natural light.

➤ Accept that it may take a few days for your child to adjust to the new time schedule, and be patient.

WEEKENDS

It can be very tempting to allow your children to go to bed later at weekends. There's no school or job to get up for, so you all sleep in, which leads to later bedtimes. As well as this, family life is very different at the weekend as it is not so structured and is much more relaxed – life is not governed by the clock as it is during the week. But bedtimes are still important. If possible, however, try not to vary the bedtime by more than an hour each night otherwise your child will find it hard to adjust again to the normal weekday routine when it's Monday morning again. If your child does have a late night, then try and wake them up at the usual time in the morning. If they are tired the following day, then you can let them go to bed earlier at night rather than sleeping in late in the morning. You may find it helps to plan things to do in the morning at weekends so that your child has a reason to get up and then enjoy the time you have in the evening after your children have gone to sleep at their normal time.

NAPTIME

The standard pattern for daytime sleep in this country is as follows: newborn babies, up until the age of about six weeks, sleep equally during the day and the night. Gradually as they get older, we teach babies to sleep longer at night with shorter and shorter sleep times during the day until daytime sleeps or naps are phased out completely. Most children under the age of 12 months take 2 naps a day – usually one in the morning and another in the afternoon. By 18 months, most have given up the morning nap but still need an afternoon kip. At age 4, more than 50 per cent of children are still taking naps because they are unable to go for a whole day easily without a rest, but by the age of 6 less than 10 per cent of children in this country sleep during the day.

There are many variations regarding the timing and length of children's naps and at what age children stop napping too but, after many decades of research, there is no agreement amongst the professionals as to which method is the best sleeping arrangement for children, or which way promotes the most restful night's sleep. In Italy, for example, the frequency of naps drops off sharply with less than 10 per cent napping at the ages of 4 and 5. In the US more than 50 per cent of children are napping at this age. In Iceland children stop napping at the age of three. Ethnic and racial factors also influence napping. In the US, studies show that between the ages of two and eight, African-American children are more likely to continue napping at older ages than Caucasian children. And in a recent study of Saudi school-aged children, up to 45 per cent of 6–13-year-olds nap on weekdays for an average of 95 minutes. The following advice on daytime naps for children is based on what seems to fit best into our northern European culture and lifestyle.

BENEFITS OF NAPPING

What research has proved is that a nap during the day, correctly timed, will promote better sleeping habits. Without a daytime nap to refresh them, many preschool children will become either progressively more whingey and irritable or hyperactive, which makes it more difficult for them to settle down to sleep at night-time. Of course, every child is different and, if a preschool child is getting the full amount of sleep they need at night, sleeping for a whole 12 –13 hours in one block, then they may not need a sleep in the day. But if they don't get their 12 hours, then ideally they should make up the shortfall during the day.

Total amount of sleep isn't the only reason children need naps though. Younger children are less able to stay awake for long periods than adults, so they need to break up their day with sleep.

Nap Benefits

➤ Contrary to popular belief, daytime naps that are properly spaced can improve night-time sleep. Sleep begets sleep.

➤ As we've seen in Chapter One, getting enough sleep is vital for the development of the brain. Dream sleep in particular, which is responsible for memory consolidation and helps children to absorb new information, occurs during daytime napping and so helps children's concentration and learning.

➤ Children and adults have a natural dip in energy in the middle of the day which coincides with a slight drop in body temperature as part of the body's circadian rhythm, making children, even good sleepers who are well rested, feel sleepy.

➤ During the day the stress hormone, cortisol, increases, and taking a nap helps to allow these levels to drop. Children who sleep during the day are able more easily to deal with daily stresses and tensions.

➤ Daytime naps refresh children so that they feel happier and more alert and can maintain their energy and focus.

➤ Children's moods will be more stable if they nap and it will even improve their appetite. A tired child who has not had a nap is more likely to become fussy and refuse food at dinnertime.

Many parents believe that allowing their children to nap during the day will make it more difficult for them to get to sleep at night or that they will not sleep for long enough at night. This can certainly be true if naps are taken at the wrong time of day. A long nap or a nap that is taken too late in the day may give your child a second wind which means that they are not tired at bedtime. However, naps will only negatively affect the length and timing of night-time sleep if they are not planned properly. If you are careful about the timing and spacing of daytime naps, your child should in fact be able to sleep better at night and therefore learn more effectively too.

HOW LONG SHOULD A NAP BE?

It is difficult to be precise about how many hours of naptime a child of a certain age needs as all children have different needs to some extent. A lot will depend on the age of the child as well as the total amount of sleep a child has in a 24-hour period.

➤ A toddler aged between 1-3 needs between 12-13 hours sleep a day plus a couple of naps
➤ A preschool child aged between 3 and 5 needs a total of between 10-12 hours sleep plus a nap
➤ A child of 5-12 also needs between 10-11 hours sleep a day and no nap. Some five year olds may still need a nap but not be able to take one because of school, in which case you should try an earlier bedtime.

So, a toddler that sleeps 13 hours at night may only need very short naps, while another child of the same age who sleeps only 10 hours at night may need to sleep for two hours during the day.

The aim of the nap is make sure your child has enough rest during the day to provide the energy they need to make the most of the day. Generally speaking it is better for children to have fewer naps but longer ones than a lot of short naps. A nap of 30 minutes, for example, is not long enough to complete a sleep cycle, so therefore most children won't benefit from a nap this short.

Help Your Child Nap For Longer

➤ Make sure your child has eaten some lunch before you put them down for a nap but don't let them have too much to drink or they may wake up needing the loo or having wet the bed.

➤ Put your child down for a nap in a dark room with no daylight coming in.

➤ Read to or with your child before the nap.

➤ Make sure your child is comfortable in bed and that they don't get too hot. Take off any jumpers and any other clothes that may cause overheating or irritate in bed.

It is, of course, much easier to prevent a child from napping too long by waking them up than it is to make a short napper sleep for longer. A nap of two to two and a half hours is about the longest you should let your child nap for. There are two reasons for this:

➤ A nap that is longer than two and a half hours may leave your child feeling groggy and disorientated when they wake up and they may cry and take a while before they are fully alert again. This feeling of disorientation won't last long but it is an indication that your child has slept for too long.

➤ If you let your child sleep for too long in the afternoon – especially if it is later in the afternoon – then your child is less likely to want to go to sleep at bedtime and less likely to get the right amount of night-time sleep.

NAP SPACING

Early afternoon from around noon to 2 p.m. after lunch is the best time for a single daytime nap because it takes advantage of your child's natural dip in energy and biological rhythm. This is the time that your child is most likely to feel sleepy even if they deny it vigorously. Not many young children will admit to being sleepy or needing a daytime nap as they are far too interested in what is going around them – there's a whole world of more fun things to do than sleep! So within that early afternoon window, it's important to watch for the signs that your child is tired and ready for their nap. For example if your child becomes quieter or alternatively more fussy and whiny and prone to tantrums, or they start rubbing their eyes and yawning (see Chapter One), you know that your child needs to be put to bed for their nap and will be likely to fall asleep quickly.

Experts recommend that you should leave at least four hours between the end of your child's nap and their bedtime. It's common sense really that if you put a child down to sleep at four o'clock in the afternoon and they sleep for two hours until six o'clock they are not going to be ready for bed again an hour or so later at seven or seven thirty. Although it is virtually impossible to stop a tired child from going to sleep at four o'clock or whenever it is if that's what they need to do, if you have scheduled your child's nap for earlier in the afternoon they shouldn't feel tired until it's their natural bedtime.

To help maintain a regular nap schedule, treat naptime a bit like bedtime and have a consistent routine that you use each day. Your child will come to predict when it's time to go to sleep after lunch and may do so more happily when they know what's coming. Try not to let your child be too energetic before naptime and introduce a quiet time before the nap begins. Read your child a story or two, draw the curtains and maybe play some quiet music if that helps.

UNSCHEDULED NAPS

It is not always possible to stick to a nap schedule, especially if you have more than one child, and you can't become a slave to your children's nap habits. There are always going to be times either when your child misses their usual nap or that they take a nap that you haven't planned!

Missing the odd nap should not cause any problems. If your child is unable to have a sleep during the day, then you may need to give them a slightly earlier bedtime than usual, but most children can accommodate this occasionally without difficulty.

More problematic is when your child falls asleep when you don't want them to! A car journey or ride in the pushchair is a very common time for a child to have a quick snooze and, no matter how hard you try to keep them awake by singing or pointing out interesting things to look at, a child determined to sleep will sleep. The trick is to be organised about this. Instead of being frustrated that your child has fallen asleep in the car just before lunch and the usual naptime, try to use car journeys to your advantage. If you know you have to make a trip, try to arrange it for when your child's usual naptime is and make your child as comfortable as you can in their car seat.

WHEN TO STOP NAPS

Studies show that many children stop taking naps at around age four, but some children will be ready to give up their nap before then and others may need a nap for longer. Some children may need a nap on some days but not on others. A child that falls asleep easily at naptime still needs it but it's important to look out for the signs that tell you when your child is ready to stop their nap:

➤ your child is consistently fidgety and restless at naptime
➤ your child takes more than 20 minutes to go to sleep at naptime or doesn't fall asleep at all
➤ your child goes to sleep easily at bedtime and stays asleep without problems through the night
➤ your child remains energetic and even tempered throughout the day and doesn't show any signs of tiredness at the usual naptime

Even when your child does give up their daytime nap they can still benefit from a period of quiet time. Use the time after lunch when they normally had their nap as a time to look at books or do puzzles or some other less active play which will restore their energy and liveliness in much the same way that a nap did.

Your child's ordinary bedtime ritual may also be broken at weekends because somebody different may put them to bed. Perhaps your child is having a sleepover at a friend's house, or you are going out and a babysitter or grandparent puts your child to bed. In the next chapter I will talk about how children react to different people tucking them in at night and how to make the process as easy as possible.

EIGHT

Bedtime Tucker-Inners and Companions

Who puts your child/ren to bed in your house? Once upon a generation ago, the answer would almost certainly have been 'mum'. The typical picture of a family looked like this: a mum who stayed at home to look after the children while the father went out to work, perhaps coming home in time to kiss the children good night. But that was about the extent of Dad's involvement in his children's bedtime ritual. Dad's role was to pay the bills while it was mum's role to pay attention to the children and their needs.

Today we live in a very altered society where it is much harder to paint a picture of a 'typical' family – every family is different. In some families both parents may work long hours, in others the mum may go out to work while the dad works at home or stays at home to look after the children. In other families parents may work part-time so that mum is home one day and dad the next. There are part-time families too – with more than a third of marriages ending in divorce, many children spend their time alternating between their mum's house and their dad's house, or they are brought up by a single parent. What this change in the way we live our lives means, among other things, is that the pattern and rules of bedtime that were set by our parents do not work for many parents today. It is not just Mum who puts the children to bed; it may be Dad or Granny, the nanny (or 'manny' as the increasingly popular male nanny is known) or the babysitter. Children may have to get used to a number of different people being responsible for tucking them into bed and turning out the light. Whoever puts your child to sleep, what is important is communication, cooperation, coordination and consistency. To make this as easy for your child as possible it's important to think about the different people who will be involved in helping your child get to sleep at night, to think how your child may respond and to have a plan in place. Empower your child by getting them involved in the process as much as possible.

MUMS AND BEDTIME

Mums have always come in all shapes and sizes but this is perhaps more true now than it's ever been before. The role of the mother is far less rigidly fixed than it was a generation or so ago. Some mums go back to work immediately after maternity leave, some mums will take a career break for their children, others will try and work flexibly or part-time. Some mothers will have help looking after their children either from their partner or family or paid help. Others may bring up their children single-handedly. There is no one right way of being a mum. What is right is what works best for you and your family. But at the same time whatever choice you make needs to take into consideration the impact on your child/ren and this includes bedtime. Bedtime rituals will be important no matter what your circumstances are but how you implement these will vary according to your lifestyle.

THE WORKING MUM

Children's bedtimes can be very difficult for mums who work long hours in the office and are trying to juggle work and home life, especially if they have a long commute to work. It's difficult to be consistent about bedtimes if you're reliant on an unreliable public transport system, and when there's always the possibility of the urgent memo/phone call/meeting in the workplace that delays the time you get home from work. This may mean that mums don't get home until quite late and yet, at the same time, many mums who haven't seen their children all day very much want to be there to put their children to bed and to spend a bit of time with their children before bedtime. This is certainly true for me. As a working mum I realistically get home around 7 p.m. As I walk through the door I am greeted with a big 'MUMMY!', which simply makes me melt. I know that it is close to his bedtime and that we really ought to be having quiet time, but an extra half hour of playtime with Mummy here or there won't do him any harm ... and anyway I haven't seen him all day! Before I know it, time has raced by and it's way past my son's healthy bedtime of 7.30 p.m.

So what are we working mums to do? In the end, I think it comes down to common sense. Your child's needs must come first. If your child needs 10 or 11 hours' sleep to function properly and to develop his full potential, then they should have this whether or not you're able to be back in time to supervise bedtime. By keeping your child up later so that you can see them, when they are not able to make up the hours in the morning is not being fair to your child. Look at the pattern of your work routine and look at what time you are able to get home. Perhaps you can make it for the last part of the routine – someone else, such as the childminder, nanny,

Dad or grandparent, does bathtime and gets your child into pyjamas and their teeth brushed and you read your child a story before the lights are turned out. If you can do this every night – or at least most of the time – and your child settles easily then this is great. But if your pattern is unpredictable, or your child is overexcited by your return from work at the last minute and finds it hard to settle to sleep knowing you're home, it is better to allow someone else to put your child to bed. If you can't be there for the evening, then make sure you can be there in the morning before you go to work and before your child goes to school or day-care so that you still get a shared time each day together during the week.

Try not to feel guilty if you are not able to be with your child at bedtime. If your child knows that you won't be there in the evening but you will be there in the morning, and if your child knows that at weekends you will be there for them, they will have that security and comfort. What will make them feel far less secure is never knowing whether you will be back in time for bedtime or not. Make a plan and stick to it so your child knows what to expect. Remember that you as a parent also have needs. This may mean that in order to be a fulfilled person you need to work and this is what enables you to be a happy parent. Better to be a happy parent who can give quality time than a resentful one who gives a lot of anxious, angry time.

THE SINGLE PARENT

If you are a single parent who does not have a partner or a support network to share the responsibility of childcare, and who is working hard during the day to make ends meet, it is perhaps particularly important that the bedtime ritual works well. You may feel you are running on empty. You are Mum and Dad so, not only are you being psychologically stretched, you are being physically tested too. At the end of an exhausting day, every parent needs to have some time to sit down and relax, but this is especially true if you are having to cope with work and childcare on your own. When you say good night to your child/ren you want to be confident that they will stay in bed and fall asleep happily and not be up and down the stairs like a yo-yo extending the bedtime for longer than your patience can bear. The key, again, is a good routine at bedtime where your children know that bedtime means just that: a time when they stay in bed and sleep.

You may find that it helps to reinforce the bedtime ritual with a reward chart. Write down all the things your child needs to do before bedtime and award a star for every night that your child completes all these activities and stays in bed after the lights have been turned out. At the end of the week, you can count how many stars have been awarded and prepare a reward for the number of stars achieved. Continuing the bedtime theme, you could end up with a full moon if your child has managed to stay in bed every night that week and have a special treat such as renting a DVD, or a trip to the leisure centre. It doesn't have to be expensive, but it should be something that motivates your child to want to stay in bed.

The reward for you will be obvious – you will have some time in the evening for yourself, even if it is just going to bed without interruption. On top of that, by helping your child to stay in bed and get the full night's sleep they need, you will be helping them to feel better during the day, study more successfully at school and be happier overall.

THE STAY-AT-HOME PARENT

No one is pretending that parents who stay at home to look after their children while they are small have any less work to do than those who go out to work but the stresses may be different. A parent who has decided to devote their time to the care of their children has a full-time job and, just as in any other chosen career, wants to make a success of it.

Part of that success is ensuring a happy and healthy bedtime and if battles occur at bedtime or the children have problems falling asleep this can be particularly upsetting for parents who are working so hard to ensure their children's needs are met. Some may feel that, because they are at home, they must be available for their children at all times and many choose to stay with their child until they fall asleep – in fact, among parents of preschool children half the parents in a recent survey reported that they have to be present in the room while their child falls asleep. And more than a quarter are still staying in the room at least once a week by school age until their child is asleep. But, once your child associates going to sleep with you being there, it can create problems if, for any reason, you are not able to be there. Your child will not be able to sleep without you. I would urge any parent to think carefully about the reasons they are staying with their child to get them to sleep. If it makes you feel happier and you can consistently do this, then fine. But it is not essential for a child's sense of security and feeling of being loved to have you in the room when they go to sleep. A happy bedtime ritual that allows you plenty of time to share with your child and tell them how much you love them, followed by hugs and kisses before you turn the light out and leave the room gives your child just as much security and teaches them how to sleep on their own, which is invaluable for the times when, like it or not, they may have to do without you.

DADS AND BEDTIME

While there are now far more dads involved in the care of their children than used to be the case a generation ago – latest figures reveal that 200,000 British men now stay at home to look after the children – it is still the case that many dads work long hours and are not able to get home early enough to help with the bedtime ritual. Just 3 per cent of fathers read to their children compared to 89 per cent of mothers. What often happens is that dads arrive home just as the mum or other carer has prepared the children for bed, calmed them down at the end of a busy day and made them feel drowsy and ready for sleep. Suddenly Dad appears and all thoughts of going to sleep disappear as the children jump out of bed for a hug or playtime with Dad. It can then take an extra half an hour before your child is ready for sleep again, or your child may miss his/her sleep window, become overtired (see Chapter Two) and not get off to sleep for some time.

Just as for the working mum, dads need to be aware of the child's bedtime ritual. It's important that parents discuss and agree what this routine is going to be so that the minimum of disruption occurs to your child's sleep habits. If Dad can consistently get home early enough from work to take part in the bedtime ritual then that is ideal. It helps the mother and the child and is rewarding for the dad too. But if the dad's working pattern is unpredictable it is better to time things so that the arrival home does not impact on the children's bedtime. Again, dads can be there in the morning or make weekends Dad's special time for putting the children to bed. Consistency, consistency, consistency!

MUMS AND DADS IN DIFFERENT HOUSES

What happens when children have two homes with different routines? About a third of children will have parents who no longer live together and who divide their time between their parents' homes. One or both of the parents may have remarried and started a second family with different rules, routines and habits. And of course this can be confusing, unsettling and difficult for children who find that the security of their world has been shattered. Sleep is often affected and children can find it hard to adjust to sleeping in different rooms in different homes. But with careful thought and preparation things can be made easier. Ideally, divorced parents are still able to agree on what is best for their child and set aside any personal differences to provide a stable routine that is followed in both households. However, this may not be possible and, if this is the case, then you will have to help your child accept that different routines occur in different houses. Again, drawing up a chart can be very helpful. Have one chart for the routine in Mum's house and another chart for the routine in Dad's house. Write down all the different things that happen in each house and when they will be doing them and on which days. For example, on Tuesdays and Wednesdays at Dad's house, share bath with step-sibling, watch TV, lights out at 8.30 p.m. On Mondays, Thursdays and Fridays with Mum, no TV after 6.30 p.m., shower, storytime, lights out at 8 p.m.

That way a child will know to expect the differences that occur at bedtime and it can make bedtimes a lot easier.

GRANDPARENTS

While many grandparents are not able to see their grandchildren as much as they would like because they are separated by distance or economic factors, many grandparents are involved in the care of their grandchildren to some degree and this can be a hugely rewarding experience for both grandparent and grandchild.

Grandparents are a link to a family's culture, history and traditions and can play a very important role in a grandchild's life. But, as with all family matters, it is important for parents and grandparents to communicate well so that no misunderstandings or resentments occur. For example, the way you discipline your child may be very different from the way you were disciplined by your parents when you were young.

Grandparents, traditionally, like to spoil and indulge their grandchildren. Parents may be surprised to see how much more relaxed and lenient their parents are towards their grandchildren than when they were brought up. Part of this may be explained by the fact that grandparents don't have to worry about how their grandchildren turn out – that is the responsibility of the parents, so surely a little spoiling can't do any harm. Grandparents are less emotionally involved. They may also get tired more easily and for these reasons manage things differently.

Getting the balance right between encouraging the bond between grandchild and grandparent, while at the same time imposing some limits on the 'spoiling' of routines can be a tricky one. You don't want to offend the grandparents but at the same time you do want to ensure that your child's routines are not always broken by grandparents who think that they know best! If the grandparent is going to help with your child's bedtime on a regular basis, it is important that you sit down and discuss the routine with them beforehand and explain why it is important that this is kept. Talk through all the details and don't think that, just because they looked after you, you don't need to clarify things. Don't make any assumptions. You may be able to include a special grandparents' bedtime treat in the routine, such as an extra story, but the basic routine does have to be kept.

Other practical considerations also need to be taken into account depending on the age of the grandparents and their physical abilities. Does the bedtime ritual usually involve a lot of physical ability – say, lifting a young child in and out of the bath – and is this fair? Do you need to subtly adjust the routine for the grandparents? If grandparents are going to put the children to bed in their own home rather than yours, make sure their home is child-safe.

Finally, make sure you can talk to your parents, the grandparents, honestly and openly about the routine so that no misunderstandings occur.

Grandparent Tips

➤ Remember that children are easily adaptable. Children will quite easily accept different styles of discipline and understand that different rules apply depending on whether they are with you or with their grandparents. Provided that you consistently enforce your basic rules, your children will accept this.

> ➤ If you are concerned that a grandparent's discipline is damaging to your child (either because it is too harsh or too indulgent) you need to say so. Explain, for example, that you do not allow your children to have a sweet before they go to bed and ask them not to do so either without directly criticising them.
>
> ➤ Get grandparents involved and ask them for help in the way you like to look after your child so that they can understand how your approach works.
>
> ➤ Remember that the love grandparents can give their grandchildren is a wonderful thing and you know that ultimately you all want the same thing: healthy, happy and rested children and grandchildren.

NANNIES AND BABYSITTERS

It can be hard for you the first time you allow someone other than yourself or a close member of the family to put your child to bed. And unless you have made careful preparations beforehand it can also be difficult for the nanny or babysitter, who will be hoping for a quiet night.

It is really important that your child has had a chance to get to know the person who is putting them to bed. If you are employing a nanny to look after your child while you are at work, try and make sure that, for the first few days at least, you are at home in time for bedtime so you can show how the bedtime ritual should work. If you're using a new babysitter, arrange a few visits first before you leave the babysitter in charge at bedtime. Show them the ropes and give them a list of ways to deal with your child in a variety of scenarios. For example: 'If Molly goes downstairs to turn on the TV after bathtime, remind her that she is not allowed to watch TV and take her back upstairs to her room', etc. Your child will feel much happier with a familiar person and more likely to settle down to sleep, which will make it easier for the babysitter or nanny too.

Talk to your child beforehand to explain that you will be going out for the evening but that you will be back when they've gone to sleep and you'll see them in the morning.

Don't expect a Mary Poppins who can magically achieve bedtime calm if you have not been able to achieve this yourself! The nannies who appear on television shows to sort out bedtime chaos are not the norm.

Do have a bedtime ritual in place. Discuss the details of the bedtime ritual carefully and write it down. This will help avoid any misunderstanding and prevent a clever child from trying to persuade the babysitter that 'Mummy says we always bake a cake before bed so it's ready for breakfast!' or 'I'm allowed to stay up until nine on Thursdays' when their bedtime is really eight!

If your child is not used to being put to bed by a babysitter, then prepare your babysitter for the possibility that your child may become upset at bedtime when the realisation dawns that they will not see you. Suggest distraction by offering another story. Alternatively, a babysitter's reward chart can work well. For each stage of the bedtime ritual successfully completed without a fuss (brushing teeth, staying in bed after lights out), the babysitter will put a sticker on the chart which the child can proudly show mum and dad in the morning.

Make sure your babysitter has all your contact details in the event of an emergency.

WHEN DO YOU STOP TUCKING YOUR CHILD INTO BED AT NIGHT?

There will come a time when your child no longer needs to be put to bed by you or anyone else. When that time is will depend on you and the personality of your child. According to National Sleep Foundation's 2004 Sleep in America poll, only 12 per cent of school-aged children put themselves to bed. Gradually, as children get older they no longer need to be reminded to brush their teeth or to go to the loo before they hop into bed and are read to. The routines they've been following will have become automatic and a habit. Nevertheless, many children like it when their parents come and say good night to them in bed, even if they don't actually need it to help them sleep. You may be surprised to find that even teenagers can secretly like it; at least if you go upstairs to say good night you are giving your child the opportunity to talk to you if they want to, and unburden themselves if there is anything worrying them which is keeping them awake.

BEDTIME FRIENDS

Most children are social creatures who like to be with other people. The presence of others is comforting and reassuring whereas the thought of being alone, especially at night-time, can be particularly worrying. There are some exceptions of course, children who – like adults – feel the need to have their own space, to have somewhere to escape to to be away from people. But most children would much rather share their bedroom with someone – or something – than go to sleep in a room on their own. Many children will share a bedroom with a sibling, not necessarily because they have to but because they find it easier to sleep at night knowing there is someone else in the room. One of my friends lives in a seven-bedroom house with four kids but all the four kids share a room because they want to. Some children will share a room, or even a bed, with their parents, and this is becoming an increasingly popular method of sleeping (see below). Children who don't have siblings to share with and don't share with their parents may create an imaginary friend who is very real to them and who can help them to sleep at night. Here's some advice on helping your child to sleep happily and safely with these bedtime friends.

CO-SLEEPING

The practice of co-sleeping, where parents share their bed with their child for as long as their child wants to, is a practice that is as old as parenting itself and one that until Victorian times was considered quite normal in this country. Then in the nineteenth century popular opinion changed and it was believed that the best way to bring up an independent child was to separate parent and child and to train children to sleep alone in a separate room from a very early age. Today in the Western world the majority of parents still follow this method. But in many other parts of the world co-sleeping is widely practised, and our method of sleep training is thought to be cruel and harmful to the child.

While for many years, the subject of children sleeping with their parents was taboo, attitudes are beginning to change. More and more parents are deciding to sleep with their babies and children and passionately believe that it helps their children not only to sleep better but to feel happier and more confident in their day-to-day life. Various studies seem to bear this out, indicating that children who sleep with their parents are less likely to be afraid of sleep and more likely to have better long-term emotional health, including being happier and less anxious and with lower stress hormones.

Those who argue against co-sleeping, and I am one of those people, believe that it can put too much stress on the relationship between husband and wife. Not having a bed to yourselves makes an intimate relationship not impossible, but more difficult. Unless a child has been through a traumatic experience and temporarily needs the comfort and security of sharing their parents' bed, I personally believe that parents need to have their own space and not having it in the bedroom may have a negative effect on the whole family. I also believe that children need to learn how to sleep alone and that this is best and most easily done for everyone concerned from the very beginning.

However, the decision whether to co-sleep with your child or not is a very personal one. If you do decide to co-sleep it is very important that you do so safely.

Safe Co-sleeping

➤ Never co-sleep if you smoke, or have been drinking alcohol or used any drugs or medications.

➤ Don't sleep with your child if you are suffering from sleep deprivation yourself and find it difficult to wake up. You should be sensitive to your child's needs.

➤ Being overweight can pose a risk to a toddler if you are likely to roll on top of them. Check the mattress for any dips, which might make you more likely to roll towards your child.

➤ Make sure your bed is safe for your child. Consider sleeping on a mattress on the floor or putting rails around the bed to prevent a young child from falling off the bed.

➤ Make sure there is no space between the mattress and the wall where your child could get wedged in.

➤ Remember that co-sleeping will add warmth so you need to be careful your child doesn't overheat. Blankets should not be too heavy or thick and pillows should not be too deep or soft to avoid the possibility of suffocation.

SIBLINGS

If you have more than one child, it can often make sense to put the children together in one room, not just because it saves space but because it can really help to bond the siblings together. Of course there will be times when the children fight, and there will be times when the children keep each other awake at night, but on the whole siblings who share a room fight less and sleep better than children with separate bedrooms, and co-sharing siblings end up with very firm friendships in place.

There are some practical things to consider. From adolescence onwards, most children tend to want to have their own rooms, or at least their own private area, which is not shared. This is particularly true for different sex siblings, although there is no law that says that brothers and sisters may not share a room over a certain age. Primary school siblings are usually happy to share bedrooms whether same sex or not.

When putting more than one child to bed at bedtime, you need to think particularly carefully how you will manage the routines so that your children all get to sleep well and you are not spending the whole evening putting different children to bed. As far as possible, try and coordinate the children to do the bedtime activities at the same time – it helps if your children are close together in age – such as sharing a bath, putting on pyjamas at the same time and brushing teeth together. You will have to work out whether you make the children go to bed at the same time or whether the older child is allowed a later bedtime. If this is the case, and they are sharing a room, they will need to learn to be quiet when going to bed so as not to wake their younger sibling. If you do put your children to bed at the same time, you might allow the older child to keep their bedside light on to read for longer. See what works best with your children – it may involve a bit of trial and error.

If your siblings share a room and they just won't wind down, separate them. When you notice your kids are keeping each other up, calmly but firmly enter the room and give one warning. The second time, enter the room and move the good sleeper to a special treat room to sleep. The bad sleeper needs to learn to sleep in their own room.

IMAGINARY FRIENDS

A child who does not have a sibling to share a room with may well invent one – or if not an imaginary sibling they may invent another invisible friend, which might be human or might be an animal. Some parents worry that this means their child has no real friends, but this is not the case. Approximately 65 per cent of young children befriend imaginary companions, and nearly one-third continue to play with them through to age 7, new research shows. Studies also show that children who make up friends tend to be more articulate, more creative and have a higher sense of self-esteem. It is healthy for children to have imaginary friends and it allows them to see things from other people's perspectives.

Children use imaginary friends in a number of different ways. They can help children deal with boredom, children can talk to these friends about things that are worrying them or use them as a voice for their concerns (my friend is worried about schoolwork ...). An imaginary friend will always do what they're told and behave in the way your child wants them to, which can boost their self-confidence especially when the friend is usually less pretty, less sporty and generally less able, but ever loyal and always there for your child when needed. Typically, girls choose younger imaginary friends and boys choose older macho friends.

So, if you hear your child talking to someone in the bedroom who you can't see, there is no need to be alarmed. If the imaginary friend, be it a tiger or a rabbit or a little girl or boy, helps your child to feel more confident, less lonely and more comforted, then your child is more likely to sleep well at night. And an imaginary friend is much easier to have for sleepovers! (But do remember to explain the presence of the imaginary friend to a babysitter or grandparent if they are responsible for putting your child to bed.)

PETS

Many children like the idea of having a pet that sleeps in their room. A cat or dog that sleeps on the end of the bed provides companionship and warmth, or at least that's the theory. Furry animals can often seem to children like wonderful soft toys that move. But real animal friends that share your child's bedroom may be more of a problem than imaginary ones. Furry animals can be a major cause of asthma – as many as 30 per cent of asthma sufferers are allergic to at least one or more animals. Although animal hair itself does *not* cause allergies, it can collect mites, pollen and mould that do. And any animal that lives in a cage, from birds to gerbils, will produce droppings that can attract mould and dust.

The advice from animal welfare groups is that preschool children should always be supervised around any animal so they certainly should not have one sleep in their bedroom. As adorable as kittens and puppies are, they are not advisable for children under five, whose loving hug may seriously injure them.

Animals such as hamsters make good pets but they tend to sleep a lot during the day and come out at night, which does not make them suitable for bedrooms.

Low-maintenance pets such as goldfish can have a therapeutic effect for older children and these make good bedroom companions. But you need to be fastidious about cleaning the goldfish tanks, or teaching your child to clean them, because the smell of a dirty tank does not aid sleep.

Although childhood pets are a wonderful source of learning and comfort and often become important members of the family, my advice would be to keep them out of your child's bedroom and to encourage your child to make a bed for their pet in another room in the house or outside.

As in all things, consistency when putting your child to sleep is important, whether it's you, your partner or the grandparents. Ensuring that your child knows the bedtime ritual, and that it does not deviate too much from place to place or person to person will mean that their good sleep habits are not broken. But what happens when you go on holiday, to a very different, unfamiliar place? I will deal with this issue in Chapter Nine.

NINE

Travelling and Other Sleepy Places

Getting your child to sleep easily and well at home and in the comfort of their own bed and familiar surroundings is one thing, but what about all the times that they are not at home or the usual routine is disrupted? Whether it's staying in a hotel on holiday, or staying at a friend's house for a sleepover there will be lots of times your child will need to learn to sleep in a different environment from the one they are used to and where they may need help getting to sleep. When travelling to these places, perhaps on a plane or in the car, getting to sleep may not be the problem but sleeping comfortably and safely may be more of an issue. You need to be flexible in these situations, and allow for the possibility that your child will find going to sleep in a new environment difficult. Here are some things to think about when travelling with your child and sleeping away from home.

SLEEPING ON THE MOVE

CARS AND CAR SEATS

There is something about the motion of the car and the low hum of the car engine that makes a sleep in the car almost inevitable for children at some point or other. Even quite short journeys can send babies and children to sleep within minutes. In fact, I know parents who, bleary-eyed from lack of sleep, put their child in their car at bedtime and drive them until their child is lulled to sleep (hoping there won't be a red light at the traffic lights to stop the car and wake the child) as they don't know any better way of getting their child to sleep. But not all children find the car easy to sleep in. Depending on how your child reacts to car journeys try and plan your trip to fit in with your child. If they sleep well in the car, then it makes sense to drive on a long trip when your child would normally sleep if you can arrange this. If your child finds it hard to sleep in the car, then plan the journey for during the daytime and provide them with lots of toys and things to occupy them, such as books, music or story CDs, or portable DVD players.

Whether you are on a long journey or a short trip you need to think about how to make your child as comfortable as is safely possible in the car – safety is obviously the most important factor in a moving vehicle. This means that you need to check that your child's car seat is appropriate for the age and weight of your child and that you are using it properly. A car seat can only protect your child if it's being used properly – it's no good loosening the straps on your child's harness to help them sleep better as you will be putting them in danger of injury in the case of an accident.

So when buying a new car seat, do talk to the shop assistant about the most suitable one for your needs. Car seats are divided into different categories depending on the weight of a child. Rearward-facing seats, which can only be used in the back seat, provide greater protection for a child's head, neck and spine than forward-facing seats but by the time your child is three years old they will almost certainly be heavy enough to qualify for the forward-facing car seats that are suitable typically for children over nine kilograms. There are lots of different types of seat available – if you and your children spend a lot of time in the car then you may want to look at the seats that recline into more comfortable sleeping positions. Forward-facing car seats can be used in either the front or back seat of the car but it is generally speaking safer to have them in the back and never put them in the front if your car has front passenger air bags.

Modern booster seats are designed for children between 15 and 36 kg (33–79 lbs) roughly aged between 4 and 6. Booster seats and booster cushions do not have an integral harness but are held in place by the car seat belt which goes around the child and the seat, so it's really important to make sure the seat belt is properly adjusted. The belt should be as tight as possible with the lap belt over the pelvic region, not the stomach and the diagonal strap resting over the shoulder and not the neck. When children first move out of the forward-facing child seats into booster seats and cushions, ones with backs may provide a better fit for the seat belt. Booster seats with side wings will also help to prevent injury in a side impact by protecting a child's head as well as making it more comfortable for them when they do sleep. Additionally, you can buy specially made car seat sleeping pillows that prevent your child's head from falling to the front or the side.

Car Journey Tips

➤ Dress your child in clothes that are comfortable for travelling and sleeping. If the journey is going to involve driving through the night, try and incorporate the bedtime ritual as far as you can. Stop for supper at their usual mealtime and then change your child into their pyjamas or usual night clothes. Play some soothing music in the car or a story CD and don't forget to bring your child's favourite bedtime toy or teddy.

➤ Arrange as many comfort breaks and stops as you can throughout the journey. The longer your child is strapped into the seat the more restless they become, and forcing a child to wait to go to the bathroom may result in an accident that is unpleasant for everyone. Other stops just to allow your child to run around will help your child to release pent-up energy and will make it easier for your child to sleep when the time comes.

➤ Try not to let your child eat junk food on the journey or food that has a high-sugar content which can increase fidgeting and hyperactivity. Pack nutritious snacks such as vegetable sticks or cubes of cheese so they have something to munch on when they are hungry.

➤ Pack sleepy snacks which may help your child go to sleep (see Chapter Ten).

➤ Don't forget to pack things that will make the journey more comfortable: toys, books and activities so your child has something to do while they're awake in the car; and blankets and things to snuggle when your child is ready to sleep.

When your journey is over, never ever leave a sleeping child (or an awake one for that matter) alone in a car even for a minute. There are so many things that could go wrong, particularly in hot weather, as it only takes a little time for a car to become like an oven and for the child to become seriously ill from heat exhaustion and dehydration. Not only that but a child who wakes up alone in a car may be frightened – especially if it takes you a while to realise that your child has woken up. Alternatively, a child may be curious and if they can get out of their car seat by themselves, get into all sorts of dangerous trouble by playing with things in the car. If you have finished your journey and your child is still asleep you can either stay in the car with them until they wake up (make sure you've got a good book to read or something else to do while you're waiting) or, if it's night-time, carry your child inside and hope they will continue their sleep without waking up.

HOLIDAYS AND SLEEPING ON AN AEROPLANE

Going on holiday with the children should be a joy and particularly if it's a big family holiday trip abroad you want to make sure you all enjoy it, but travelling with the children can be a challenge too. If your children don't sleep properly while you are away, or the journey is fraught from lack of sleep, then you will all end up being exhausted rather than relaxed and refreshed as holidays are meant to make you feel. However, with a bit of planning and preparation beforehand you can avoid some of the problems that can occur from sleeping away from home.

ON THE PLANE

Much of the advice for sleeping in the car can be applied to sleeping on a plane: make your child feel as comfortable as possible and disrupt routines as little as possible.

➤ If you are going on a long flight, try and schedule the journey to fit around naptime or bedtime and make sure that your child has lots of opportunity to use up physical energy before they have to sit on the plane for hours.

➤ Most children will want to sit next to the window so that they can see out. This also has the advantage of ensuring less distraction from the flight stewards and passengers walking up and down the aisles.

➤ During take-off give your child something to suck on or give them a drink from a sippy cup (you can take liquids on board a plane provided you buy the drink after you've been through airport security) so that their ears are not affected by the change in cabin pressure. Drinking milk can have a mild sedative effect too and is comforting. Talk to them about what is going to happen and reassure them if they find the noise of the engines frightening.

➤ Once the plane has taken off and your child has had a chance to look out at the clouds, pull down the window shutter and turn off the overhead lights.

➤ Dehydration can be a real problem for children in planes. Encourage your child to drink regularly. Not all airlines have water that is suitable for drinking so it's best to take your own drinking water with you in your cabin bag.

➤ Go through as much of your child's sleep routine as possible, including putting on pyjamas, reading books, letting them listen to quiet gentle music and giving your child their favourite bedtime toy. Most airlines will be able to supply blankets but, if you have space to take them on as hand luggage, your child's own blanket and pillow may help them to sleep much more comfortably.

SEDATION

Some parents may be tempted to ask their GP for a sedative to help their child sleep on long plane journeys or to buy over-the-counter medication. While the idea that giving your child something to make them sleep soundly for the whole journey may sound appealing – and is in fact quite widespread – most experts would not recommend this. For one thing these drugs can have side effects such as respiratory problems. For another, the antihistamines contained in the drugs can also have the opposite effect of making your child sleepy and cause children to become overexcited and less controllable. This state may last several hours before it wears off and, while not medically dangerous, will make your journey far, far worse than it might otherwise have been. As a final warning, experts say that if a child is sedated and their airways become blocked, by a nose pressed against a seat for example, their natural reflex to shift position may be blunted. Instead, doctors recommend that for children who find it difficult to sleep on aeroplanes it is better to make sure that they are well rested before the journey and that they have something to keep them occupied during the flight like a small toy or a book. And finally, and most importantly, don't consider sedating yourself either with alcohol or medication – you will not be in a fit state to look after your child properly.

JET LAG

Travelling across time zones and the resulting disruption to our sleep–wake cycle which we call jet lag can be hard for both adults and children. While the body clock resets itself and tries to adjust to the new time, you and your children may experience tiredness, trouble sleeping and headaches. Especially if your holiday is not long, you want everyone to recover from the change in time as soon as possible so that precious days of your holiday are not wasted by everyone feeling tired, out of sorts and irritable.

How to Overcome Jet Lag Easily

➤ Get on to the new time and reset your watches as soon as you arrive – or even before you arrive, while you're travelling. Try to keep your child awake until the local bedtime, don't let them nap in the late afternoon however much they want to, and wake them up the next day at the local morning time. Give meals at the new time too.

➤ Keep your child hydrated with as much water as possible and encourage them to eat juicy food which will hydrate too, like fruit and vegetables. Eating healthy snacks without much sugar should help too.

➤ Go for a walk. The daylight and the fresh air will help your child adjust to the new time and the exercise will help your child's body cope too. Also, the excitement of the new surroundings will prevent your child from wanting to go to sleep at an inappropriate time.

➤ Remember to pay attention to the direction of travel and when your kids sleep. Travelling east causes the most jet lag because this is when you lose time. If you are travelling west and gaining time your child may have trouble falling asleep that first night. Provide a dim light and allow them to do a quiet activity like reading a book or playing with their toys until they do fall asleep but wake your child up at the local time the next morning even if they went to sleep much later than normal.

> ➤ Make sure your child eats enough during the day so they don't get hungry during the night. Don't let them sleep through meals and skip eating anything.
>
> ➤ Eating at the local time is a good way to help reset the body clock.
>
> ➤ Don't be tempted to use sleep aids such as sleeping pills to help your child sleep. Your child's body clock needs to learn to adjust to the new time change naturally. And many pills have the effect of making children feel more alert and hyper than sleepy.
>
> ➤ Be patient! Your child's body clock (and yours) will reset but it may take a day or two to get used to the new rhythm.

IN THE HOTEL

The excitement of being on holiday coupled with being in an unfamiliar environment where everything, from the food to the language and scenery and the beds, is different can make sleeping difficult even for children who normally have no problems at bedtime. While part of the point of going on holiday is for our children to experience different cultures and surroundings, to help your child sleep as well as possible try and make some things as much like home as you can.

Bring familiar things from home with you to make their temporary sleeping environment comforting. Although space is a problem when packing, you might like to bring your child's pillow because the familiar smell can aid sleep and because hotel pillows can often be uncomfortable. If your child has a comfort blanket don't forget that or a bedtime toy, as well as a few of their favourite bedtime books. If your child is old enough, get them involved in packing for the trip so that they can choose what most precious things they want to have with them.

In the hotel room, try creating a space for your children to play in where they can get out all their toys and re-create their home environment. Pack things like a night light if that is what your child is used to. It will help if your child does wake in the middle of the night because you won't have to turn on the main lights – and fully wake your child as well as everyone else – and means everyone can find the bathroom in the middle of the night. It makes it easier for your bedtime too, allowing you to read before you go to sleep if that's what you're used to.

Try and stick to the usual bedtime rituals as much as is possible and give your child time to wind down at the end of the day. Especially if you've had a busy schedule of sightseeing or other activities your child will need to have time to settle down before they are ready for sleep. If your itinerary permits, you may want to begin the bedtime ritual slightly earlier than you would normally to allow for a longer settling period before sleep. If there is a TV in the hotel room, your child may find this very exciting but try not to let them watch it before bed; have the usual bath, story, lights out routine instead.

Safe Sleep

When you're sleeping away from home with young children, the first thing you want to check is that the bedroom or sleeping environment is safe for your child.

➤ Look at the furniture and where it's placed and if there is anything you're worried about, such as a bed not being pushed against a wall, or a headboard with a cut out area which your child might get their head stuck in, ask if you can move things to your satisfaction. Don't leave heavy suitcases on luggage racks which can be pulled over by young children and cause injury. Check that beds are not too close to the window or near window blinds, cords and curtains, and that night lights lamps and electrical items are away from where your child sleeps.

➤ Make sure you know where the fire exits are.

➤ If there's a mini fridge in the bedroom, make sure that any alcohol is kept well out of reach or see if it's possible to lock the fridge.

➤ Check the bedding. While most hotels will wash the sheets on the beds after each guest checks out, most only wash the bedspreads occasionally. Bedspreads can be home to all sorts of germs as a result so it's best to remove them, especially as they will often make your child too hot in bed anyway. Bring your children's mattress and pillow protectors. They are easily portable and don't take up much luggage space so you can take them on holiday with you and know that your children will have a fresher and more hygienic night's sleep.

➤ Wipe down surfaces with disinfectant wipes. According to some research in the US, viruses can be found on almost every surface in hotel rooms such as door handles, TV remotes, light switches, taps and so on. There are a variety of disinfecting wipes on the market so to prevent your child from getting ill (and the inevitable sleep disruption that goes with illness) wipe down these items in hotel rooms to get rid of any harmful germs.

SLEEPOVERS

There will come a time, sooner or later, when your child begs and begs you to allow them to have friends over for a sleepover, or to be allowed to go to a sleepover at a friend's house.

And there will come a time when you have to say 'yes'! Now part of the point of a sleepover is that children don't follow their usual bedtime ritual. They do not go to bed at the normal time, they do not eat the usual sensible food and they do get to watch a DVD, eat popcorn and stay up chatting with their friends. So there is no point in trying to insist on the usual bedtime rules. However, in order for the sleepover to be successful and for everyone to enjoy themselves, you do need to establish some rules and help the children to get some sleep.

HOW OLD DO YOU NEED TO BE?

The first thing is to be as confident as you can that your child and their friends are old enough to be able to enjoy a sleepover properly. There is no set age that children need to reach before taking part in a sleepover as each child is different and will be ready for one at different ages. But, if your child finds it difficult to sleep without a particular routine or has other sleep problems such as waking in the night or bed wetting, it is better to wait until your child is older before taking part in a sleepover.

HOSTING A SLEEPOVER

Whatever your child tells you, sleepovers work much better if there aren't too many people. One or two at the most is ideal and definitely only one person the first time you and your child host one.

The probability is that the chosen friend/s will already have been to your house for tea or a play and so will know the layout and where to find things, but if this is not the case then give them a guided tour so they know where the loo and the bathroom is and where they will be sleeping.

Get the child/ren to set up their sleeping bags. If there are not enough beds for everyone, it's best if everyone sleeps on the floor to prevent any disagreements about who sleeps where.

Talk to the friends' parents first and check that they've told you everything you need to know: any allergies, anxieties, special things needed at bedtime, etc.

Have some activities up your sleeve in case the children get bored or don't know how to occupy themselves (see overleaf for ideas). Encourage some outdoor fun for as long as possible or until it gets dark so that they tire themselves out, but be prepared to take part in board games or cooking or whatever the children enjoy doing.

Get the children changed into their pyjamas and then let them snuggle up on the sofa to watch a film (which you've checked isn't scary or upsetting first). Give them popcorn and hot chocolate to drink but not too many sweets or they'll be far too wired to go to sleep later. If they still want things to munch, prepare a plate of fruit like banana, strawberries, mango, melon and kiwi all cut up and arranged beautifully and see if this tempts them.

Stick to the bedtime you've agreed they can stay up till and not later. Turn the lights out but let them talk and laugh for quite a while afterwards. If they are happy they will eventually fall asleep. If, however, the friend gets a bit tearful, try and reassure them first and let them phone home if necessary. If this doesn't help, you may need to arrange for their parents to come and collect them.

Be prepared for the children waking up early in the morning even if they've stayed up much later than normal the night before. Set a rule about what time they are allowed to get up, and be ready for a noisy breakfast! Make sure you've got a variety of cereals and perhaps a breakfast treat like pancakes or pain au chocolat.

Fun Sleepover Activities

➤ **Scavenger hunt.** Hide things in the garden for the children to find – small wrapped sweets, bouncy balls, glitter nail polish, temporary tattoos, stickers, etc. A night-time scavenger hunt can be even more fun – the children each have a torch and have to find things in the dark. This can be done inside too if the weather is bad.

➤ **Pillow painting.** Get a set of fabric paints and let the children design their own funky pillowcase which they can take home.

➤ **Talent contest/charades.** For sleepovers with several friends, these activities are great fun.

➤ **Storytelling.** Once the lights are turned out, the children can take it in turns to tell each other a story – either one that they've made up, or a familiar story with a twist.

➤ **Cooking.** Buy pizza bases and let the children add their own toppings: ham, pineapple, peppers, pepperoni, cheese, tomatoes, sweetcorn, etc.

➤ **Make a mummy.** Using a toilet roll, one child wraps the other one up in toilet paper to make a mummy. Messy but fun!

➤ **Two truths and a false.** Friends take it in turn to tell each other facts about themselves and get the friend to guess which 'fact' is false.

While consistency is important in your day-to-day life in order to foster good sleeping habits for your child, do remember that you need to be flexible when your child is put in a strange and unfamiliar environment. By being sensitive to your child's needs, you can ensure that they still get a good night's sleep while on holiday, making the days you spend away from home together even more fun and enjoyable!

TEN

Food for Sleep

Can food help your child sleep? The simple answer is yes it can if your child is eating the right sort of food. But if your child is eating the wrong sort of food it can also hinder sleep. The busy lives we lead often means that we look for fast (and cheap) options when it comes to providing meals. We need to rediscover our common sense and realise that with food moderation and a balanced diet is essential for a healthy lifestyle.

The best food for our children is often not the easiest to prepare, can be more expensive and more perishable, but paying attention to what your child eats and the extra effort involved in providing good food is important on lots of different levels. As celebrity chefs such as Jamie Oliver have highlighted over recent years, by making a few small adjustments to what your child eats, you can have a profound effect on their health, their concentration and their schoolwork, their behaviour, their confidence and, of course, their weight and fitness levels. It can also affect the way your child sleeps (and the way you sleep too for that matter).

If your child is eating a healthy diet and sleeping well, then you have nothing to worry about. But, if your child is having problems getting to sleep or not sleeping for long enough, it may be that their diet has something to do with it.

With obesity rates on the increase we could be breeding a generation of fat, sleepless children. So it's vital that we understand how food affects the body and which foods to eat to aid sleep and which to avoid; it can make a real difference both to your child's daytime and night-time sleep.

Lora moved to a new school which was further away and meant leaving the house at 7.30 a.m. – much earlier than the 8.15 a.m departure time she was used to. Breakfast had been an important meal of the day for her, but she had to eat it on the drive into school. By lunchtime, which was at 12.45 p.m., she was ravenous and ate a double portion of chips, meaning that by the time the day was over she was looking to fill herself up on the way home, usually on junk food. By dinnertime she was again ravenous and continued to eat well into the evening which prevented her from getting off to sleep and her weight started to increase. Over a period of three months Lora's parents noticed her mood changing, her concentration levels worsening and her schoolwork start to be affected. Her mum decided to make sure that she got up a little early to have a decent breakfast before she got in the car and that her school bag was packed full of healthy snacks such as raisins, apples and sticks of celery, carrots and cheese for her to graze on in her morning break. This meant that Lora wasn't ravenous by lunchtime. Her parents also got her to have a 30-minute walk with them after school. Dinner would consist of sleepy foods, such as turkey and mash followed by a banana and a warm drink of milk just before bedtime. Over a period of one month, as Lora's sleep improved so did her mood, along with her schoolwork and concentration levels. Sleeping better also meant that her weight started to drop as she had the energy to exercise more, at the same time as her parents made sure she was eating healthy food.

FOOD TO HELP SLEEP

Different types of food affect the body in different ways depending on what is contained in the food. Some types of food contain stimulants which will increase energy for a period of time making you less sleepy. Other types of food produce chemicals in the brain that promote calm and sleepiness. Foods that help sleep contain a substance called tryptophan. Tryptophan produces a brain chemical called serotonin from which melatonin – so essential for sleep that it's named the 'sleep hormone' – is manufactured. Studies made in 2005 have shown that people who ate foods with high amounts of tryptophan improved their chronic sleep problems within three weeks of changing their diet. Foods that are high in tryptophan include:

➤ nuts such as almonds, cashews and walnuts
➤ poultry, in particular turkey
➤ bananas
➤ dairy products – cheeses such as Cheddar, Gruyère and Swiss cheese have particularly high amounts of tryptophan
➤ green leafy vegetables such as cabbage and spinach

➤ kidney beans
➤ oats
➤ wheat
➤ eggs
➤ tofu and soya products

But in order for the tryptophan to help your child feel sleepy they need to eat these foods combined with healthy carbo-hydrates. Carbohydrates cause the release of insulin, which helps tryptophan reach the brain and cause sleepiness. Good examples of meals that combine the two foods are:

➤ turkey with a small baked potato
➤ pasta with some Cheddar cheese grated on top
➤ an egg sandwich made with wholewheat bread
➤ tofu with stir-fried vegetables
➤ tuna with salad and wholewheat bread

If your children are fussy eaters, try using your imagination to make food more enjoyable for them. Arrange the food so that it looks like their favourite cartoon character or a funny face, for example. By making your food visually appealing to your child you'll soon see that they will tuck in!

Other Good Sleep Foods

Here is a list of some other foods that are known to help sleep and which you might like to include in your child's evening meal:

Lettuce: as the Flopsy Bunnies discovered in Beatrix Potter's famous Peter Rabbit books, lettuce has a 'soporific' effect –

on children as well as rabbits! Lettuce contains a substance called lactur carium that helps promote sleep by sedating the nervous system. Its sleep-promoting properties have been well documented over the centuries – even the Ancient Egyptians used it. If you can get your children to eat salad for supper, they may sleep better.

Porridge: oats contain small amounts of melatonin, the hormone that promotes sleep. A bowl of porridge mixed with bananas and ginger, which also contain melatonin, would make a very good pudding for sleep, especially if you added warm milk and honey to it. However, melatonin is mostly flushed from the system within an hour of entering the bloodstream so your child would need to eat it about half an hour before bedtime to get any effect. Other foods that contain melatonin are sweetcorn and tomatoes.

Marmite: Marmite helps to release insulin which will help sleep, so a perfect sandwich for supper would be Marmite and lettuce on oatmeal bread.

Honey: although too much sugar is stimulating, a little glucose is thought to be helpful for sleep because it tells your brain to turn off orexin, which is linked to alertness.

Bananas: if your child was just to eat one bedtime food, then the banana would probably be it. As well as having the tryptophan, it also contains the sleep hormones melatonin and serotonin, and magnesium, which is a muscle relaxant. Bananas mashed with warm milk and honey would be a super-sleep combination.

FOODS THAT HINDER SLEEP

If your child has ever come back from a birthday party where they've eaten lots of sweets and drunk fizzy drinks and they've been bouncing all over the place, then you'll have seen first hand that there are some foods that generate energy and hinder sleep. It's unlikely they will go to sleep for several hours after eating so much of the wrong sort of food. But food affects people differently depending on their individual make up and metabolism. So whereas for some children sugar consumption can aggravate problems such as hyperactivity, anxiety, nervousness, irritability and poor concentration – all of which can lead to sleep difficulties – other children may be unaffected.

The fact is, though, that for the majority of children the food that tends to have the worst effect on sleep is the type of food that many children are particularly attracted to: sugar, cakes, fizzy drinks, tomato ketchup, baked beans, sweets, pastries, white bread, rice and pasta, all of which contain refined sugar. Once digested, the sugar shoots into the bloodstream giving your child an instant high. When this departs from the system the body craves another sweet fix to feel energised again. A continued cycle of sugar highs and lows can cause hormonal imbalances, weight gain and sleeping problems. Limiting the amount of refined sugar your child eats is sensible for a healthy diet anyway, but when your child does have a meal that has lots of sugar, try and make sure that it's several hours before bedtime so that the effects of the sugar rush have worn off.

Foods that are high in protein also generate energy and wakefulness, particularly if they are eaten on their own without fat or carbohydrates, so you should avoid giving your child a high protein meal before bedtime. Examples of high protein foods to avoid include red meat, bacon and pork, ham and sausages.

Sleep problems can also be caused by foods that act as stimulants and foods that cause indigestion and gas.

➤ Spicy food and acidic food, such as orange and grapefruit juices, which can cause heartburn. Lying down makes heartburn worse, and the discomfort from heartburn hinders sleep.

➤ Fatty, greasy or rich creamy food, which again can cause heartburn and indigestion.

➤ Caffeine. You may know that caffeine is a stimulant which keeps you awake but think that as your child probably doesn't drink coffee you don't need to worry about it. But caffeine can be found in much less obvious sources including chocolate, cola drinks and tea. Beware of coffee-flavoured food too, such as yoghurt or ice cream – coffee-flavoured yoghurt can contain as much caffeine as a cola drink. Many energy drinks contain guarana, a natural source of caffeine that contains more milligrams of caffeine per ounce than coffee. Some medicines also contain caffeine, including many daytime cold medicines, so it's worth checking the labels of your child's medication. For better sleep for your child, avoid giving them any caffeine after lunchtime. Don't be too worried, however, if you give your child cocoa before bedtime. A cup of hot chocolate barely reaches 5 mg of caffeine, compared to instant coffee, which contains approx 60–80 mg of caffeine, and a freshly ground cup of coffee, which contains 90–150mg.

FOOD SENSITIVITY, INTOLERANCE AND ALLERGY

Allergies are very common in children and it is estimated that up to 40 per cent of children have an allergy to one type of food or another. The first sign that your child is allergic to something may be that they are not able to sleep well. Allergies cause the nasal tissues to swell and to secrete excess mucus, which means they may suffer from a night-time cough, snore loudly, have a stuffy nose or have difficulty breathing at night. The common foods to cause sleep problems in children who have allergies are dairy products, eggs, nuts and wheat. If you recognise any of these symptoms in your child and think they may be allergic it's best to visit your GP before eliminating the food from your child's diet.

ADDITIVES

Artificial food additives such as preservatives, colours and flavours, sweeteners and thickeners which are added to improve the taste and appearance of processed food are found in many foods that are eaten by children, including breakfast cereals, sweets and drinks. Although the E number given to each food additive proves that it has been scientifically tested and approved as being safe to use in food in Europe (hence the E), for some years there has been controversy over whether there is a link between additives and hyperactivity in children. There are many parents who believe that E numbers do have an effect on some children's behaviour making them hyperactive, restless and disrupting their sleep patterns.

In the UK, The Food Standards Agency recently funded research into the subject by the University of Southampton. The study looked at the effects of different 'cocktails' of drinks containing artificial food colours and other additives in 153

3-year-olds and 144 8- and 9-year-olds from the general population. Teachers and parents were asked to keep a diary outlining their children's behaviour changes after they drank the 'cocktails'.

The results suggested that parents are right – some food additives do cause hyperactivity in some children – and this can cause sleep problems not just in children who already suffered from being hyperactive. The children who consumed drinks with colourings were more likely to have tantrums, become restless and be prone to allergic reactions. The advice from the Food Standards Agency is that, while it's important to remember that there can be many factors that contribute to hyperactive behaviour in children, if your child shows signs of hyperactivity you might choose to avoid giving your child food and drinks containing the following artificial colours:

- sunset yellow FCF (E110)
- quinoline yellow (E104)
- carmoisine (E122)
- allura red (E129)
- tartrazine (E102)
- ponceau 4R (E124)

These colours can be found in a wide range of brightly coloured foods including some soft drinks, sweets, cakes, jelly, jam and ice cream. Check the food labels if you want to avoid these foods. If you buy any foods that are sold without packaging you will need to check with the person selling the product or with the manufacturer.

TIMING OF MEALS – GOING TO BED
ON A FULL TUMMY

Many families today have their main meal in the evening. Children often take packed lunches to school, and parents grab a sandwich in their lunch hour, whereas in the evening there is more time to prepare a cooked meal and to sit down as a family to eat it. Unfortunately this is the opposite of what we ought to be doing to get the best night's sleep. When your child eats, as well as what and how much they eat, has an effect on how well your child sleeps. If your child has a big meal just before going to bed their metabolic rate and body temperature will increase instead of decreasing which will make it harder for them to get to sleep. The expert advice is that midday is the best time to eat a large meal and to have a small meal or snack in the evening. Children (and adults) need energy during the day not at the end of it when they are going to sleep and their body should be resting not digesting. However, if for practical reasons you need to give your child their main meal in the evening, try to make it as early in the evening as possible before their bedtime and at least two hours before they go to sleep.

At the same time, being hungry can keep children awake as well. A small bedtime snack eaten about half an hour before bedtime can solve the problem. Bearing in mind the foods that help sleep, here are some suggestions for good bedtime snacks:

➤ porridge with bananas
➤ wholegrain crackers with tuna or Cheddar cheese
➤ yoghurt and low-sugar muesli
➤ turkey sandwich with cheese on wholemeal bread

➤ peanut butter sandwich
➤ a warm milky drink and an oatmeal biscuit

FRESH FOOD AND EATING HEALTHILY FOR HEALTHY SLEEP

The government is campaigning hard to promote the importance of eating five pieces of fruit and vegetables a day – the 'five-a-day' message has been widely advertised in the media for a number of years now. Nevertheless, there are still many children who aren't getting enough fresh food in their diet and this affects their general health, including their sleep. A healthy diet that includes lots of fresh food including fruit and vegetables, rather than processed food, will help promote sleep because these foods release energy slowly, which balances blood sugar levels and sustains energy without hunger pangs.

Ensuring your child's diet is full of fresh whole foods will also help prevent your child from eating too much salt, additives and preservatives, which are often found in ready meals and processed and refined foods. Too much salt can lead to high blood pressure in later life and, as we have seen, additives and preservatives can act as stimulants and stop your child from having a good night's sleep.

It's not always easy getting children to eat healthily. Some children are very picky eaters and it can be difficult to make sure these children get enough variety in their diet. Interestingly research suggests that being a fussy eater is an evolutionary trait: children who are fussy about eating tend to be fussy about the same types of food – meat, fruit and vegetables – that in earlier times were the types of food most likely to cause food poisoning. The studies suggest that parents can help a wary child to try a new food by eating it themselves first, thereby proving that the food is not harmful. Children often need active persuasion to eat food that is good for them. Food habits are formed very early in life and can be hard to changer later on so the sooner we persuade children to eat healthily the better. A generation ago, children were made to eat what was put in front of them whether they liked it or not. Today, our approach is somewhat softer and we try and encourage rather than force children to eat what they're given.

Healthy Eating Tips for Sleeping Well

➤ Don't keep any junk food in the house. If it's not available, then your child can't eat it. Instead, stock your larder with healthy fruit and vegetables, such as chopped-up celery sticks and carrots, wholegrain bread, crackers and cereals. What you don't buy you don't eat.

➤ Involve your children in what they eat. Get them to help you plan the menu, take them shopping with you and talk about the food you are buying and why it will make them feel good, and let them help with preparing the food. Young children can grate the cheese, or mash the carrots, for example. Older children may like to try cooking a whole meal. I know it can be stressful having to deal with the mess that results when children help you cook, but if it helps your child to eat well and sleep well, in the end it will be less stressful and worth it.

➤ As often as you practically can, sit down as a family to eat a meal together. You can act as a great role model for your children if you demonstrate how enjoyable it is to eat a healthy meal. If you are eating the green vegetables and the fruit, you may be able to persuade your children to eat them too.

➤ Plan a menu that contains a variety of food, experiment and be adventurous. Prepare food in different ways – for example, a child who doesn't like roast parsnips may like them when they're mashed, or those who refuse to eat mushrooms in a salad may happily finish a bowl of mushroom soup.

➤ Don't force a child to eat something they really don't want to eat, but encourage a child to try something new with a reward chart. Every time a child tries a new healthy food they can put a sticker on the chart. When they have got enough stickers, they can be rewarded with a treat such as a trip to the swimming pool or ice rink.

➤ Talk to your child about food, help them understand how their body works and why it is important for them to have a mix of carbohydrates, proteins, fats, vitamins, minerals and fibre to grow and develop healthily.

NUTRIENTS FOR HEALTHY SLEEP

A healthy diet should include all the nutrients necessary for your child to function properly and that includes sleep. The following nutrients have been shown to be natural relaxants and are particularly important for healthy sleep:

B Vitamins: these are most closely linked to a good night's sleep and the control of tryptophan, especially vitamin B3 found in lean meat, oily fish, wheatgerm and dried fruit; vitamin B6 found in whole grains, wheatgerm, bananas and walnuts; and vitamin B12 found in dairy products, eggs and lean meat.

Iron: low levels of iron have been associated with some sleep problems such as restless legs syndrome. To make sure your child has enough iron in their diet, you can give them spinach, lean meat and poultry.

Magnesium and calcium: a deficiency in these minerals has also been associated with waking during the night. Sources of magnesium include bananas, wheatgerm, nuts, seeds and wholegrains, and sources of calcium include dairy products and green leafy vegetables.

Zinc: this is known to promote restful, restorative sleep. Sources include dairy products, oats and pumpkin seeds.

MIDNIGHT MUNCHIES

Although rare, some children suffer from a sleep-related eating problem called night eating or the 'Dagwood' syndrome. Children with this problem typically are unable to get to sleep without eating at night. They don't eat anything until after midday and eat more than half of their diet at night-time.

Night eating in children may be caused by a variety of things including having an ulcer, dieting during the day, by being overstressed, by low blood sugar or by 'a routine expectation' or conditioned behaviour. This means that children don't eat at night from genuine hunger but because they have learned to expect food at this time. For example, most babies can sleep through the night by the age of six months, but some babies continue to wake through the night because when they do so they are given milk then. An older child may wake up during the night and ask for something to eat or drink refusing to go back to bed until they've eaten the snack. This behaviour will continue for as long as their requests are granted. The best treatment of the problem is for the parent to deny the request for food and drink in the night if they don't think their child is really hungry. Eventually the child will stop waking up in the night asking for food. My son has never been a great eater but has always loved his milk at night-time. Although it was difficult, I decided to withdraw his night-time milk drink. It made a massive difference and he was subsequently more interested in food during the day.

OBESITY AND SLEEP

The relationship between food and sleep in children is an intricate one. As we have seen, what children eat can have an effect on how they sleep but, equally, how well children sleep and how long they sleep for has been shown to have an effect on children's weight. In several studies over the past few years, a link has been found between sleep deprivation and the increased risk of obesity in both children and adults. One study in 2006 which looked at over 28,000 children found that infants who slept less than 12 hours a day ran almost twice the risk of becoming overweight preschoolers. The recommendation of the experts leading the trials was that parents should use sleep hygiene techniques (e.g. bedtime rituals) to improve the length of time their children slept for in order to prevent them from becoming overweight.

More research is needed to understand the reasons why lack of sleep can lead to obesity. One theory is that a child's appetite is increased as a result of hormonal changes caused by lack of sleep. It is also possible that mothers tend to use food to settle wakeful babies. Other factors include lack of exercise and too much TV watching. Children who exercise more will need more sleep and are less likely to be obese. Likewise children who watch more TV exercise less and sleep less and this too contributes to obesity. To help children eat sensibly and improve their chances of sleeping well it's important to:

➤ ensure your child eats enough fresh, healthy food
➤ give your child regular mealtimes. Mealtimes can act as a cue to sleeping patterns. If a child regularly has their evening meal at the same time each night, their body will be ready for sleep at the same time too
➤ make sure your child doesn't eat a large meal too close to bedtime. There should be an interval of two hours between a large meal and going to sleep
➤ don't give your child food that contains stimulants after midday
➤ allow a small healthy bedtime snack but not less than half an hour before bedtime
➤ never use food as a comforter or a means of getting children to sleep
➤ ensure your child gets enough physical exercise every day (see page 4 for more information about this)

The importance of giving your child a healthy, well-balanced diet to set them up for the day and for their future lives is well-known, but you may not have known just how essential the right sorts of foods are for ensuring your child gets a good night's sleep. Giving your child healthy food, making sure they exercise at least an hour a day, creating a restful sleeping environment and bedtime ritual means that your child will be ready to sleep once they've been tucked in and it's time to turn out the light. And a good night's sleep means that your child will wake up refreshed and ready to take on the world.

Conclusion

'Once upon a time there was a child who was always grumpy and bad-tempered. He didn't do well at school and was always bumping into things and having little accidents. His parents were at their wits' end. Then one day the sleep fairy came to visit and waved her magic wand to make the child sleep well at night. In a very short time, the child found he could concentrate in class and started to do well at school. He stopped losing his temper (most of the time, anyway!) and he had more energy and enthusiasm for doing things in the day. He became a much happier little boy who woke up in the morning with a smile on his face. And he and his parents lived happily, ever after.'

Of course, in real life, there is no such thing as a magic wand we can wave to help our children sleep. But, as I have talked about in this book, there are things we can do to help our children sleep well at night, every night, which can almost magically transform the way our children behave and feel.

Until the age of ten, our children spend almost half their lives asleep. Although there is still much that we don't yet know about sleep, we do know that our children need sleep to grow, to learn, to behave, to be happy, to stay well and to minimise the risk of injury, and even to control their weight. In time, research will no doubt reveal even more about the benefits of sleep.

Teaching our children to sleep well from the outset by paying attention to their bedroom environment, bedtime ritual, exercise and diet is fundamental to their health and happiness. In my opinion it is more fundamental than teaching them good table manners, more fundamental even than giving them a good education; if our children aren't sleeping well they are less able to make the most of the opportunities around them or to have the capacity to take anything on board. Preventing sleep problems and teaching our children healthy sleep habits is vital for their well-being.

It is vital for our well-being too. A sleepless child means sleepless, tired and frustrated parents who may well be suffering with the same symptoms as their children: looking and feeling tired, weight gain, bad moods and no patience. The effects of lack of sleep on us as parents can affect our feelings towards our child and how we manage the problem. In most cases a child's sleep problem will pass in the fullness of time but, in the meantime, you need strategies to help manage the problem as best you can. And do not underestimate how important it is that your child sees that you, too, have healthy sleep habits. You have a responsibility to your child to establish good patterns of behaviour that will set them up for their adult life. Your child follows your example, so it's for your child's benefit – and your own – to deal with any sleep problems you might have.

In this book, I have looked at how our children's busy, non-stop, high-tech, high-speed lives lead to lack of sleep. Mental overstimulation and physical understimulation, where our children are constantly entertained and given little time to literally switch off (the remote control, the mobile phone, the computer) and unwind combines to make healthy sleep much harder to achieve.

We don't need magic to help our children sleep – a dose of common sense will often do. We need to listen to our children and to understand their concerns to help them to sleep better. We need to be consistent in helping our children develop good sleep habits and we need to pay attention to the things that we can change, such as the bedroom environment, routine, diet, exercise, and the use of mobile phones, Internet and the TV in the bedroom. If, after doing all these things, a child's sleep problem still doesn't resolve, then it is time to seek professional help.

I am not saying that if we have a child who can't sleep, we have failed as parents. Nor am I saying that you must follow an unwavering and strict regime and do exactly what I say to address problems of sleep. We all have busy lives and we need to take into account our own needs too, when working out how to help our children sleep better. There may be times when the stresses and difficulties of our lives make it difficult to provide the patience, time and consistency that help our children sleep better. Recognising this, and looking to our support network for help at difficult times – as well as being realistic about what we can and can't do – will help us to work out the best way to manage our children's sleep.

And the rewards for helping our children sleep well are huge. Not only will they benefit in all the ways we have talked about but there are few things more wonderful than looking in on your child before you go to bed and watching them while they are restfully asleep, or snuggling up to your sleepy, dream-filled children in the morning after a delicious night's sleep.

In short, sleep is an active and dynamic state, which greatly influences our waking hours, and is fundamental to our children's and to our own existence. With a healthy sleep routine your child's and your own daytime potential for health and happiness is not just a sweet dream but assured, and, after reading the guidelines in this book, my hope is that you and your children will have a 'Good night and sleep tight'.

Sleep Contacts

RESOURCES

Sammy Margo

www.sammymargo.com

Tel: 020 7435 4910

Email: sleep@sammymargo.com

Sammy Margo is a sleep expert and chartered physiotherapist available for consultation.

The Chartered Society of Physiotherapy

www.csp.org.uk

Tel: 020 7306 6666

Email: enquiries@csp.org.uk

The Chartered Society of Physiotherapy (CSP) is the professional body for the UK's chartered physiotherapists, physiotherapy students and assistants.

The London Sleep Centre

www.londonsleepcentre.com

Tel: 020 7725 0523

Clinic for diagnosis and treatment of sleep disorders for children and adults. Referral may be via your GP or direct.

Millpond

www.mill-pond.co.uk

Tel: 020 8444 0040

Provides guidance to help parents resolve their children's sleep issues and provides training to healthcare professionals.

Sleep Scotland

www.sleepscotland.org

Tel: 0131 651 1392

A charity offering sleep counselling to families whose children have additional support needs and sleep problems(18 months and upwards)

Parentline

www.parentlineplus.org.uk

Tel: 0808 800 2222

Provides free help and support for anyone in a parenting role. The service includes a 24-hour helpline.

Gingerbread

www.gingerbread.org.uk

Tel: 0808 802 0925

An organisation offering support, advice and friendship to lone parents.

Relate

www.relate.org.uk

Tel: 0300 100 1234

Provides a confidential counselling service for anyone experiencing relationship difficulties with their partner or family member.

Hyperactive children support group

www.hacsg.org.uk

Tel: 01243 539 966

Provides information for parents of hyperactive children where the hyperactivity may be related to diet or chemicals such as food, toothpaste, bubble bath, fragrances, detergents or intolerances/allergies.

PRODUCTS

SlumberSlumber

www.SlumberSlumber.com

Tel: 0800 028 1111

Provides information and reviews on products relevant to sleep for children and adults, including duvets, pillows and linens, and natural and anti-allergy options.

Abaca

www.abacaorganic.co.uk

Tel: 01269 598 491

Manufacturer of soil association certified organic mattresses in the UK. All standard sizes of mattresses as well as bespoke sizes available.

Audible

www.audible.co.uk

Tel: 0800 08 25 100

Provider of downloadable audiobooks.

SLEEP DISORDER CLINICS

Referral should be made through your GP.

Index

The Good Sleep Guide

By Sammy Margo

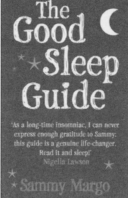

Almost a quarter of the UK population frequently experience sleeping difficulties. If you have trouble sleeping and often wake up feeling exhausted, *The Good Sleep Guide* is the answer.

This essential handbook will help you understand the importance of the right environment, look younger and feel more energised, discover the best over-the-counter sleep remedies and say goodbye to sleep disorders, such as insomnia and sleep apnoea.

With advice on the best mattress to buy, which sleep position is optimal and the importance of routine, as well as explaining why you sleep badly and what you can do about it, *The Good Sleep Guide* is a practical, accessible and lively book to help you sleep better, for good.

£9.99   ISBN 9780091923488

Order this title direct from www.rbooks.co.uk

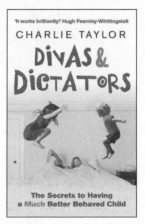

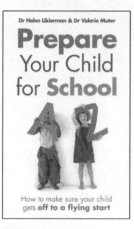